SINDA: Standardized Infant NeuroDevelopmental Assessment

T0203259

SINDA: Standardized Infant NeuroDevelopmental Assessment

An instrument for early detection of neurodevelopmental disorders

Mijna Hadders-Algra
Professor of Developmental Neurology, Department of Paediatrics, University Medical Center Groningen, University of Groningen, Groningen, the Netherlands

Uta Tacke
Child Neurologist, Neuropaediatrics, University Children's Hospital Basel, Basel, Switzerland

Joachim Pietz
Paediatrician, Palliative Medicine, Center for Child and Adolescent Medicine, Medical Faculty, University of Heidelberg, Heidelberg, Germany

Heike Philippi
Child Neurologist and Chair, Centre for Child Neurology, Goethe University, Frankfurt, Germany

2022
Mac Keith Press

Original title: SINDA – Standardized Infant NeuroDevelopmental Assessment: Untersuchung zur Früherkennung von neurologischen Erkrankungen und Entwicklungsstörungen im ersten Lebensjahr by Hadders-Algra / Tacke / Pietz / Philippi

©2021 W. Kohlhammer GmbH, Stuttgart.

©2022 Mac Keith Press

Managing Director: Ann-Marie Halligan
Senior Publishing Manager: Sally Wilkinson
Publishing and Marketing Co-ordinator: Paul Grossman
Production Manager: Andy Booth

First published in this edition in 2022 by Mac Keith Press
2nd Floor, Rankin Building, 139–143 Bermondsey Street, London, SE1 3UW

British Library Cataloguing-in-Publication data
A catalogue record for this book is available from the British Library

Cover designer: Marten Sealby

ISBN: 978-1-911612-61-2

Typeset by Riverside Publishing Solutions Ltd
Printed by Hobbs the Printers Ltd, Totton, Hampshire, UK

Contents

Foreword

The Standardized Infant NeuroDevelopmental Assessment (SINDA) is clinical developmental neuroscience at its best: intellectually sharp, child-fitting, and methodologically in-depth. It covers the early life span between 6 weeks and 12 months and brings together all relevant dimensions of development.

Using the neurological, developmental, and socio-emotional scales, SINDA covers the infant's bio-psycho-social complexity from the beginning.

After the introduction, background, and psychometric properties, the reader is led systematically through an infant-adapted neurological scale that covers motor function, cranial nerves, muscle tone, and reflexes/reactions. The developmental scale uses monthly steps to carefully describe what to look out for and what this tells you about infants' eye-contact, imitation, exploration, object manipulation, etc. The socio-emotional scale adds interaction, emotion, regulation, and responsiveness/reactivity. Every item is described precisely, and most are accompanied by photographs and wonderful to watch video sequences.

SINDA allows for accurate detection of infants at high risk of developmental disorders, making it a valuable tool for doctors, students, paediatric neurologists, developmental specialists, psychologist, and therapists alike. As comprehensive as SINDA is shown to be, are there areas that could be improved in the future? The answer is both no and yes. No, with regard to completeness, clarity, photos, videos, and all the wonderful easy-to-understand and easy-to-use material. Yes, with regard to the clinically driven wish to turn to a 'short version' to make it even more user-friendly in the real world of clinical settings and challenges.

As the title suggests, with this book, an updated 'new' standard instrument is given for the first 12 months of a child's life and it invites you and your colleagues to update yourself, your institution, your team, and your co-workers to follow and observe one of the most fascinating stages of growth: early human development.

Let me strongly recommend SINDA by paraphrasing a well-known saying: 'if you want to improve something, measure it'.

Florian Heinen
President of the German-speaking
Neuropaediatric Society (GNP),
Munich, Germany

Preface

This book is a practical guide on the Standardized Infant NeuroDevelopmental Assessment (SINDA). SINDA is a neurodevelopmental assessment for infants aged 6 weeks to 12 months corrected age and aims to detect infants at high risk of neurodevelopmental disorders. Health professionals will be able to use SINDA on the basis of this manual, thanks to its many illustrations and its over 160 accompanying video clips. No additional instructional course is required.

The book contains the following information: Chapter 1 introduces SINDA's three scales: the neurological scale, developmental scale, and socio-emotional scale. It highlights that the scales do not only serve early detection, but also parent counselling. Chapter 2 discusses the dynamic developmental changes in the young brain and the risk factors of atypical neurodevelopment. The chapter stresses two important consequences of the rapidly developing brain: (1) early detection of high risk of neurodevelopmental disorders is challenging, but certainly possible and (2) early detection is needed in order to be able to exploit the young brain's high plasticity by means of early intervention. Chapter 3 addresses the design, the practical implementation, and the excellent psychometric properties of SINDA.

Chapters 4 to 6 form the main body of this SINDA guide: they contain the standardized description of all items, including information on the infant's position, the procedure required to assess the item, and the criteria for typical and atypical performance. Chapter 4 presents the 28 items of the neurological scale. Chapter 5 describes the developmental scale. This scale is organized by age in months: it contains 15 items per month. Chapter 6 addresses the six items of the socio-emotional scale.

Chapter 7 discusses the significance of the findings of the three SINDA scales. It addresses which scores are considered as atypical and what further actions are required in infants with atypical scores.

The work described in this book is the result of the collaboration and contribution of many people. We gratefully acknowledge the enthusiastic support of Professor Florian

Heinen, MD, during the final phases of the completion of the SINDA manual. We thank the interdisciplinary team of the SPZ Frankfurt-Mitte for their sustained interest in SINDA and the energy to collect the data of our clinical samples. We also thank the physiotherapeutic team of the University Children's Hospital in Basel, Switzerland, who successfully motivated their patients' families to participate and to provide video recordings of their infants. We are especially grateful for the wonderful and skilled assistance of Anneke Kracht who produced all the figures and video clips. We also wish to express our sincere thanks to André Rupp, PhD, for his great statistical support. We thank Donna Tennigkeit (medical student) for entering the clinical data into the data files.

The collection of the Dutch normative data would not have been possible without the contribution of colleagues from the KinderAcademie in Groningen (heads: Selma de Ruiter, PhD, and Francien Geerds, MSc), that of many medical master students, and that of Ying-Chin Wu, PT, PhD, and Patricia van Iersel, PT, PhD. Last but not least, we thank the many parents and infants who participated in the studies underlying the SINDA manual, in particular those who allowed us to use images (figures and/or video clips) of their infants to illustrate SINDA.

The collection of the normative data was part of the IMP-SINDA project that was financially supported by the Cornelia Stichting and the Stichting Ontwikkelingsneurofysiologie Groningen. Finally, we acknowledge the technical assistance of Linze Dijkstra with the IMP-SINDA project.

Mijna Hadders-Algra, Uta Tacke,
Joachim Pietz, and Heike Philippi
December 2021

Videos

The supporting videos and materials are available to those who have purchased the book or been given access by Mac Keith Press. Please follow the below steps to access the supporting material.

A. I have bought the book from Mac Keith Press directly at www.mackeith.co.uk

1. If you have bought the book directly from Mac Keith Press, you can access the supporting materials by clicking on "MY ACCOUNT" / "LOG IN OR REGISTER" in the upper-right corner of the web page. You must be logged in with the account with which you bought the book.
2. Then, click on "Memberships" from the list of options.
3. Next, click "VIEW" on SINDA: Standardized Infant NeuroDevelopmental Assessment (Supporting Materials).

Alternatively, you can use this direct link if you are already logged in: https://www.mackeith. co.uk/sinda-standardized-infant-neurodevelopmental-assessment-supporting-materials

B. I have bought the book from another source or third party

Those who have purchased the book from a third party may still access the videos by sending a request with proof of purchase to admin@mackeith.co.uk. Once your request has been processed, you will be able to access the supporting materials using the steps outlined in A.

[Some items are marked with a red dot (●), which indicates that the item involves interaction and that the item is also used to assess 'interaction' of the socio-emotional scale.]

Video 4.1	Assessment of SINDA's neurological scale in an infant aged 5 months in supine position
Video 4.2	Assessment of SINDA's neurological scale in an infant aged 9 months
Video 4.3	Varied and symmetric movements of arms and hands in an infant aged 4 months (Items 2 and 3)

## CHAPTER 1

Introduction

WHAT IS SINDA?

The Standardized Infant NeuroDevelopmental Assessment (SINDA) is a clinical screening instrument to detect infants at high risk of a developmental disorder. The early detection of high risk facilitates the provision of optimal family guidance. SINDA can be used in infants aged 6 weeks to 12 months corrected age. SINDA has been designed for professionals involved in the early detection of developmental disorders, for instance paediatricians, developmental paediatricians, child neurologists, paediatric physiotherapists, occupational therapists, and speech therapists. It is an instrument that provides health professionals not only with information on the infant's current neurodevelopmental status but also with information on the infant's risk of developmental disorders, such as cerebral palsy, intellectual disability, or behavioural disorder (Hadders-Algra et al. 2019, 2020).

SINDA consists of three scales:

- *The neurological scale*: 28 items with criteria that are similar throughout the age range of 6 weeks to 12 months. Special attention is paid to the quality of spontaneous movements. The scale takes about 10 minutes to complete.

- *The developmental scale*: only the 15 items corresponding to the infant's corrected age need to be completed. There are 113 items altogether in the developmental scale covering the entire age range. The items address cognition, communication, and fine and gross motor development. The time needed to perform the developmental scale is age-dependent; it varies from 5 to 7 minutes in the youngest infants to 10 to 15 minutes in the oldest infants.

- *The socio-emotional scale*: evaluates four types of behaviours: interaction, emotionality, self-regulation, and reactivity. The items are identical for the entire age range. They are evaluated during the assessment of the neurological and developmental scales, and take no additional assessment time.

SINDA can be performed in virtually any environment. It requires simple equipment, consisting, for instance, of a mattress and some attractive objects that can be purchased in any toyshop, e.g. a small Mickey Mouse puppet, a rattle, and a ball.

WHY SINDA?

SINDA has been developed because a concise instrument that evaluates the infant's neurological, developmental, and socio-emotional status did not exist. Of course, instruments that address a single domain are available. For instance, the infant's neurological condition can be evaluated with the Hammersmith Infant Neurological Examination (HINE; Haataja et al. 1999; Romeo et al. 2016), and with the methods of Amiel-Tison (Amiel-Tison and Grenier 1986) and Touwen (Touwen 1976). From these methods, the HINE is most frequently used internationally and is quickest to perform. However, the HINE pays only limited attention to the quality of spontaneous movements, whereas the scientific literature stresses the importance of the quality of spontaneous movements to assess the integrity of the infant's brain (Touwen 1990; Michaelis and Berger 2007; Heineman and Hadders-Algra 2008; Berger and Michaelis 2009; Hadders-Algra et al. 2010). We therefore gave the quality of spontaneous movements an important place in SINDA's neurological scale. Another disadvantage of HINE is that its criteria for 'at risk' are age-dependent and not available for all infant ages.

The most commonly used instruments to assess the infant's developmental and socio-emotional status are the Bayley Scales of Infant and Toddler Development (Bayley 2006), the Griffiths Mental Development Scales (Green et al. 2015), and the Mullen Scales of Early Learning (Mullen 1995). These instruments are full assessments, whereas SINDA aims to screen the infant's condition. In comparison to the full developmental tests, SINDA: (1) has the shortest age span – it focuses on the first year of life; (2) is the quickest to complete; (3) is easier to learn; (4) is cheapest as its testing material consists of common toys and objects that can be easily purchased (Hadders-Algra et al. 2020).

This means that SINDA is the only instrument that is able to screen the infant's neurological, developmental, and socio-emotional condition relatively easy and at little cost. It is an instrument that can be integrated without difficulty in the clinical routines of health care professionals involved in paediatric care.

THE SINDA MANUAL

This SINDA manual explains the application of the SINDA scales. Chapter 2 is a theoretical chapter that summarizes the developmental processes occurring in the young human brain. This forms the basis to discuss the challenges in the early detection of developmental disorders and the need of early intervention. Chapter 3 describes the practical requirements to perform SINDA and provides information on SINDA's psychometric properties.

Chapters 4 to 6 form the core of the manual, they describe the method of testing of each item and the criteria for typical and atypical performance. Chapter 4 addresses the neurological scale, Chapter 5 the developmental scale, and Chapter 6 the socio-emotional scale. The chapters are not only illustrated by figures, but also by many video examples, that are available online (see access details on page xi). Chapter 7 discusses the interpretation of the three SINDA scales in terms of the risk of developmental disorders and the need for early intervention.

Finally, two practical remarks. First, the infant ages used in this manual always refer to ages corrected for preterm birth, unless otherwise indicated (e.g. fetal ages and gestational ages of infants born preterm). This is not further indicated in the text. Second, we use the word 'parent' not only to denote a parent of the infant, but we also use it to denote any person who accompanies the infant during the assessment.

## CHAPTER 2

Early Detection of Infants at High Risk of Neurodevelopmental Disorders

A major challenge in infant health care is the detection of infants with or at high risk of a neurodevelopmental disorder. The challenge is brought about by the amazing developmental changes in the young brain. These changes interfere with a precise prediction at early age of neurodevelopmental disorders. Yet, the young brain's high plasticity also offers opportunities for early intervention. Therefore, this chapter aims to discuss the following subjects: (1) we first review the developmental changes in the young human nervous system. Next, we summarize (2) the aetiology of neurodevelopmental disorders and (3) the challenges in early detection of neurodevelopmental disorders. We conclude with (4) a brief discussion of the need for early detection in infants at high risk of developmental disorders as it is the starting point for early intervention aiming to promote the infant's developmental outcome and family well-being.

THE DEVELOPMENT OF THE YOUNG HUMAN NERVOUS SYSTEM

The development of the human brain takes many years: it is not until the age of 40 years that the nervous system obtains its full-blown adult configuration (De Graaf-Peters and Hadders-Algra 2006; Hadders-Algra 2018a; Fig. 2.1). The developmental processes in the brain are the result of a continuous interaction between genes and environment, activity, and experience.

Neural development starts in the fifth week postmenstrual age (PMA) with the ectodermal development of the neural tube. The very young neural tube already produces

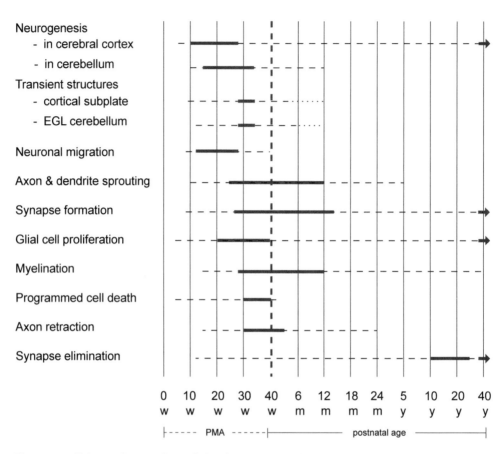

Figure 2.1 Schematic overview of the developmental processes occurring in the human brain. The bold lines indicate that the processes mentioned on the left are very active. The broken lines denote that the processes still continue but less abundantly. The diagram is based on the review by Hadders-Algra (2018a). EGL, external granular layer; m, months; PMA, postmenstrual age; w, weeks; y, years. Reproduced with permission from Hadders-Algra (2021b).

spontaneous activity. Indeed, the first fetal movements emerge at 7 weeks PMA, i.e. already before the spinal reflex loops have been completed. This illustrates that intrinsic, patterned spontaneous activity is a quintessential property of neural tissue. Soon thereafter, however, the afferent information associated with spontaneously generated movements assists the further sculpting of the brain (Hadders-Algra 2018a, 2018b).

Shortly after the closure of the neural tube, specific areas near the ventricles start to generate cortical neurons. The majority of cortical neurons are formed between 5 and 25 to 28 weeks PMA. From their origin in the ventricular layers the neurons move to their final place of destination in the more superficially located cortical plate. The process of migration is very active between 12 and 28 weeks, and it peaks between 20 and 26 weeks PMA. During migration the neurons start to differentiate, i.e. they start to produce axons, dendrites, synapses with neurotransmitters and receptors, the intracellular machinery, and the complex neuronal membranes. Remarkably, the first generations of neurons do not migrate to the cortical plate; they halt in the cortical subplate.

The cortical subplate is a transient structure between the cortical plate and the future white matter. It is the major site of neuronal differentiation and synaptogenesis in the developing cortex, it receives the first ingrowing cortical afferents (e.g. from the thalamus), and it is the main site of synaptic activity in the midfetal brain (Kostović et al. 2015). This implies that the subplate is a major mediator of fetal motor behaviour. This is illustrated by the finding that the emergence of synaptic activity in the cortical subplate coincides with the emergence of the varied and complex general movements, i.e. the movements in which all parts of the body are involved and virtually all combinations of joint configurations are tried out (Hadders-Algra 2018b).

The subplate is thickest between 28 and 34 weeks PMA. Before that age, starting at 25 to 26 weeks, subplate neurons gradually die off and later generated neurons start to populate the cortical plate. These developmental changes are accompanied by a relocation of the thalamocortical afferents that now grow to their final target in the cortical plate (Kostović et al. 2014a).

In the third trimester of gestation the cortex increases in size and gyrification starts (Kostović and Judas 2010). During this phase the subplate recedes, while the cortical plate expands. This also implies that the human cortex at this time is characterized by the co-existence of two separate but interconnected cortical circuitries: the transient foetal circuitries located in the subplate and the immature but progressively developing permanent circuitries centred in the cortical plate. The 'double circuitries' state ends when the subplate has dissolved. This situation is reached in the primary motor, sensory, and visual cortices around 3 months post-term but first around the age of 1 year in the associative prefrontal cortex (Kostović et al. 2014b).

Development of the cerebellum involves similar processes but with a different time course. Cerebellar neurogenesis peaks between 12 and 34 weeks, a period during which especially the most numerous cerebellar cells, the granule cells, are formed. The granule cells are generated in the external granular layer, another transient structure in the young brain. This layer is most clearly present between 12 weeks PMA and 3 to 4 months after term age. From the external granular layer the granule cells migrate inwards – not outwards like the cortical neurons – to their final destination in the internal granular layer (Hadders-Algra 2018a).

Brain development also involves the creation of glial cells. Glial cell production occurs in particular in the second half of gestation. Part of the glial cells, i.e. the oligodendrocytes, take care of axonal myelination. Oligodendrocyte development peaks between

28 and 40 weeks PMA (Volpe 2009). Myelination is prominently present in the third trimester of gestation and the first 6 months postnatally (Yakovlev and Lecours 1967; Haynes et al. 2005). However, myelination is a long-lasting process that is completed around the age of 40 years (De Graaf-Peters and Hadders-Algra 2006).

The development of the nervous system does not only involve the generation of neurons and connections, it also involves regressive phenomena: neuronal cell death, axon retraction, and synapse elimination. The process of neuronal death has already been mentioned. It is estimated that in the mammalian central nervous system about half of the created neurons die off through apoptosis. The neurons die as the result of interaction between endogenously programmed processes and chemical and electrical signals induced by experience (Lossi and Merighi 2003). A well-known example is the axon elimination during the development of the corticospinal tract. The tract begins with bilateral projections to the spinal cord, but gradually – starting during the last trimester of gestation – the axons of the ipsilateral projections are eliminated. The elimination process takes until about the age of 2 years, when the corticospinal tract finally consists of mainly contralateral projections (Eyre 2007). The elimination of synapses in the brain starts during the midfetal period. However, in the cerebral cortex synapse elimination is most pronounced between the onset of puberty and early adulthood (Petanjec et al. 2011).

Brain development also involves the development of neurotransmitters and their receptors. The transmitters and their receptors are present from early fetal life onwards (for a review see Herlenius and Lagercrantz 2001). Interestingly, the periterm period is characterized by a transient specific setting of various transmitter systems, i.e. by a temporary overexpression of the noradrenergic α2 receptors and glutamatergic N-methyl-D-aspartate receptors, a relatively high serotonergic innervation, and a high dopaminergic turnover. It has been suggested that this neurotransmitter setting around term age induces an increased excitability, among others expressed by the motoneurons, and that this temporary transmitter setting facilitates the transition from the fetal periodic breathing pattern to the continuous breathing needed for postnatal survival (Hadders-Algra 2018b).

In summary, during fetal life and the infant's first post-term year the brain shows high and unique, age-specific developmental activity. The most significant changes occur in the second half of gestation and the first 3 months post-term, in particular in the cortical subplate and cerebellum. As the transient subplate pairs a high rate of intricate developmental changes and interactions with clear functional activity, two phases of development have been distinguished: (1) the transient cortical subplate phase, ending at 3 months post-term when the permanent circuitries in the primary motor, somatosensory, and visual cortices have replaced the subplate; and subsequently, (2) the phase in which the permanent circuitries dominate. In the latter phase, in particular during the remainder of the first post-term year, the brain's major developmental changes consist of axon reconfiguration, dendrite and synapse production, abundant myelination, and an integration of the permanent circuitries in the association areas (Hadders-Algra 2018a).

Table 2.1 Conditions associated with neurodevelopmental disorders

Condition	Timing
• Genetic causes	From conception onwards
• Malformation of the brain, e.g. lissencephaly or schizencephaly	Prenatal: 1st half pregnancy
• Infections, e.g. CMV, chorioamnionitis, neonatal sepsis, meningitis	Prenatal, perinatal, neonatal
• Exposure to toxic substances, e.g.	
• alcohol	Prenatal
• antiseizure medication, e.g. valproic acid	Prenatal
• mercury	Prenatal and postnatal (breast feeding)
• corticosteroids	Postnatally in infants born preterm
• bilirubin	Neonatally in infants born preterm and at term
• Fetal growth restriction[a]	Prenatal: 2nd trimester (early onset) and 3rd trimester (late onset)
• Preterm birth[b]	Between 22–24 and 37 weeks PMA
• Hypoxia-ischaemia	From midgestation onwards: prenatally, perinatally, and neonatally in infants born preterm and at term

Based on Stanley et al. 2000; Mwaniki et al. 2012; Dan et al. 2014; Deciphering Developmental Disorders Study 2015; Miller et al. 2016.

[a]Birthweight <10th centile. [b]In 2014 the estimated global preterm birth rate was 10.6%, equating to almost 15 million live preterm births in 2014 (Chawanpaiboon et al. 2019). CMV, cytomegalovirus.

AETIOLOGY OF NEURODEVELOPMENTAL DISORDERS

The major groups of conditions that may give rise to and are associated with developmental disorders are summarized in Table 2.1. Whether or not a condition or risk factor, such as foetal growth restriction or preterm birth, will result in a developmental disorder depends on:

• the timing of the risk event;
• the intensity of the risk event;
• the duration of the exposure to the risk condition;
• the resilience of infant and family.

It also depends on whether the risk condition occurs in isolation or in combination with other risks. For instance, it is well known that cerebral palsy is often the result of a chain of unfavourable conditions (Stanley et al. 2000). An example of a chain of adversities is maternal smoking during pregnancy, intrauterine growth restriction, and preterm birth finally resulting in an intraventricular haemorrhage.

The risk events may give rise to malformations of the brain, to brain lesions, such as periventricular leukomalacia or an infarction in the territory of the middle cerebral artery, or to more subtle, microstructural disruptions of brain development.

CHALLENGES IN EARLY DETECTION OF NEURODEVELOPMENTAL DISORDERS

The significant neurobiological changes in the young brain have major consequences for the neurodevelopmental diagnostics in the infant's first postnatal year. In the following three sections we discuss the most important ones.

Neurodevelopmental Assessment Needs to be Age-Specific

The continuing developmental changes in the young brain invoke the need for age-specific assessments. In other words, the evaluation techniques need to be adapted to the age-specific characteristics of the nervous system. Standardized Infant NeuroDevelopmental Assessment (SINDA) is designed for infants aged 6 weeks to 12 months corrected age. We selected 6 weeks corrected age as the lower age limit, as it is the age at which the infant's brain has just passed the periterm period of transient physiological hyperexcitability. SINDA's upper age limit (12 months) has been determined by our aim to develop a neurological scale that is independent of the infant's age. In infants up to the age of 12 months it is possible to evaluate motor reactions to postural stimulation, such as the pull-to-sit or vertical suspension, in a similar, standardized way. However, from about 12 months, when infants are almost or entirely able to walk independently, these reactions can no longer be reliably evaluated. At that age the brain's capacity for anticipatory postural control has improved to such an extent (Cignetti et al. 2013) that children no longer agree to the testing of the infant motor reactions to postural stimulation.

The developmental changes determined SINDA's age range. Within the selected age range, SINDA has been constructed in such a way that (1) SINDA's neurological scale is independent of the infant's age, not only in terms of which items are tested but also in terms of the criteria for typical and atypical performance and the cut-off for the 'at risk' score; (2) SINDA's developmental scale has a different set of items for each month of age but an identical cut-off for atypical performance for each age; (3) SINDA's socio-emotional scale has identical items and criteria for atypical behaviour.

Neurodevelopmental Dysfunction is Expressed in an Age-Specific Manner

The age-dependent characteristics of the nervous system affect the way in which brain dysfunction is expressed. In adults, neurological impairment is expressed by means of specific and localized signs, e.g. in the form of the specific syndrome of a spastic hemiplegia in the case of stroke. In contrast, neurological impairment in young infants is virtually always expressed by means of generalized and unspecific dysfunction. For instance, an infant born preterm with a left-sided haemorrhagic infarction may respond with generalized hypotonia, generalized hypertonia, hypokinesia, a hyperexcitability syndrome, or with abnormal general movements (Hadders-Algra 2004; Hamer et al. 2018). In infants later diagnosed with cerebral palsy, the early unspecific signs of neurological impairment gradually develop into the specific (spastic, dyskinetic, or ataxic, unilateral or bilateral) syndrome of cerebral palsy. As a result, cerebral palsy is generally first diagnosed from about the end of the first postnatal year onwards (Granild-Jensen et al. 2015). However, many exceptions to this general rule exist. For instance, in some children the diagnosis of unilateral spastic cerebral palsy may be made in the second half of the first year, whereas in other children it may take several years before the clinical picture of cerebral palsy is fully established. Also, for other developmental diagnoses the clinical expression takes time. For instance, the first subtle signs of autism spectrum disorders generally emerge in the second half of the first year (Ozonoff et al. 2010), but the mean age at diagnosis is currently still 4 to 5 years (Zwaigenbaum and Penner 2018).

Early Prediction of Neurodevelopmental Outcome is Challenging

The marked developmental changes of the brain during the first postnatal year (Fig. 2.1) have important implications for the ability to predict the infant's risk of neurodevelopmental disorders at an early age. Infants may have had a complicated neonatal history, including a lesion of the brain (e.g. an intraventricular haemorrhage), and may present with atypical neurodevelopmental signs in early infancy. Yet, it is possible that the large neuroplastic changes during the first postnatal year induce a disappearance of the atypical performance – infants may grow out of their deficit. The reverse is also possible: children may be virtually free from atypical signs at early age, but grow into an atypical performance with increasing age due to the age-related increase in complexity of neural functions and increasing environmental demands (Hadders-Algra 2002; Zwaigenbaum and Penner 2018). The infant with an early lesion of the brain – and its associated reduced neural repertoire – gradually grows into a deficit.

EARLY DETECTION PAVES THE WAY FOR EARLY INTERVENTION

The previous section underlined that it is difficult to diagnose neurodevelopmental disorders in the first year of life. However, this does not preclude early intervention. Infants without a neurodevelopmental diagnosis, but at high risk of getting one, are in need of early intervention in order to exploit their neuroplastic potential. Early intervention does not primarily aim at treating or preventing a potential future diagnosis. Early intervention aims to assist the infant and the infant's family in the current situation of daily life. This situation is generally characterized by distress of the parents and by concerns about the infant's atypical neurodevelopment, including the infant's impaired capacities to explore the environment. Early intervention addresses both components (Spittle et al. 2015; Hadders-Algra et al. 2017; Hadders-Algra 2021a; Hadders-Algra 2021b). First, it aims to support the parents, in particular by promoting the parents' understanding of how to interact with the infant. This is especially needed when the infant has been admitted to the neonatal intensive care unit after birth. Second, early intervention also aims to promote infant development by utilizing the high neuroplasticity of early development.

What does this mean for SINDA? SINDA is a screening instrument that aims to detect infants at high risk of developmental disorders. If SINDA indicates that the infant is at risk of a developmental disorder a dual pathway is recommended: (1) further diagnostics to elucidate the origin of the infant's 'at risk' performance; and (2) the provision of early intervention. This will be further discussed in Chapter 7.

## CHAPTER 3

Design, Psychometric Properties, and Implementation of SINDA

This chapter consists of four parts. The first part discusses the design of Standardized Infant NeuroDevelopmental Assessment (SINDA), the second part describes SINDA's psychometric properties, and the third part addresses the implementation of SINDA in clinical practice. The chapter concludes with a small introduction to the following chapters that describe the SINDA items in detail.

DESIGN

SINDA is a neurodevelopmental screening instrument for infants aged 6 weeks to 12 months corrected age. It has been designed in such a way that it can be used relatively easily and quickly by professionals involved in infant health care, such as paediatricians, developmental paediatricians, child neurologists, paediatric physiotherapists, occupational therapists, and speech therapists. SINDA provides professionals not only with information on the infant's current neurodevelopmental status but also on the infant's risk of a neurodevelopmental disorder, such as cerebral palsy, intellectual disability, and autism spectrum disorder.

SINDA consists of three scales, a neurological, a developmental, and a socio-emotional scale. The design of the scales is summarized below. The items of the scales are described in the following chapters.

Neurological Scale

SINDA's neurological scale has been designed as a tool that (1) covers all infant neurological domains; (2) is standardized, i.e. has an identical set of items and criteria for infants aged 6 weeks to 12 months; (3) results in a cut-off score for those 'at risk' that is largely independent of the infant's age; (4) takes about 10 minutes to perform, including recording of the scores on the one page assessment form (see Fig. 4.1); (5) includes a substantial proportion of items evaluating the quality of spontaneous movements; and (6) assists the prediction of developmental outcome.

The scale consists of 28 items covering five neurological domains:

- *Spontaneous movements* (eight items): seven of the eight items evaluate movement quality in terms of variation versus stereotypy. The eighth item addresses the quantity of motility. The inclusion of a relatively large proportion of items evaluating the quality of spontaneous movements is based on the growing awareness that the quality of spontaneous movements reflects very well the state of integrity of the infant's nervous system (Heineman et al. 2011; Hadders-Algra 2018c). The classification of movement variation versus stereotypy is based on clinical observation, not on video assessment as in the assessment of general movements (Heineman and Hadders-Algra 2008). This implies that only striking stereotypies, including consistent asymmetries, are recorded as 'atypical'. This is in line with clinical practices (Touwen 1990; Michaelis and Berger 2007; Berger and Michaelis 2009; Hadders-Algra et al. 2010). The inclusion of seven items on movement quality also means that milder forms of movement stereotypy may be distinguished from more severe ones. For instance, the head-turn preference that is relatively often observed in young infants and may be accompanied by an asymmetry in arm and hand movements only results in a reduction of maximally three points in the domain of spontaneous movements (i.e. with a loss of less than half of the points that can be obtained in this domain; for details see below). This contrasts with the presence of markedly stereotyped movements in all parts of the body that will result in a seven-point reduction of the domain score. The latter means that the infant's score falls into the 'at risk' category (see below).
- *Cranial nerve function* (seven items): this domain includes items assessing facial and oral motor behaviour, eye movements, and reactions to light and sound.
- *Motor reactions to postural stimulation* (five items): this domain contains, for instance, the pull-to-sit manoeuvre and vertical suspension.
- *Muscle tone* (four items): this domain evaluates muscle tone in the neck and trunk, arms, legs, and feet.
- *Reflexes and reactions* (four items): this domain does not only contain tendon reflexes, but also the foot sole response and foot sole sensibility, i.e. the response of the infant's foot to gentle tickling of the foot sole.

Each item is scored as 'typical' or 'atypical' according to defined criteria (see Chapter 4). In many items the presence of a consistent asymmetry results in the assignment of 'atypical'. Addition of the item scores results in the neurological scale score. Its maximum score is 28 points; a score of ≤21 is considered to be an 'at risk' score, indicating that the infant is at high risk of a neurodevelopmental disorder (Hadders-Algra et al. 2019).

SINDA does not include responses that are clearly age-dependent, such as the Moro reflex, the palmar and plantar grasp responses, and the parachute reaction. Inclusion of such responses would have been incompatible with the age-independent construct of the neurological scale.

Developmental Scale

SINDA's developmental scale has been designed as a tool that (1) provides information on the infant's developmental status; (2) covers cognition, communication, and fine and gross motor development; (3) consists of 15 standardized items per month of age; (4) results in an age-specific score that is largely independent of the infant's age; (5) is easy to apply by professionals working in infant health care and takes relatively little time to perform; (6) assists the prediction of neurodevelopmental outcome at older age.

The developmental scale consists of 113 items that are ordered age-wise with 15 items for each month of age, starting at 2 months and ending at 12 months (each month ±2 weeks). Application of the developmental scale means that only the 15 items corresponding to the infant's corrected age in months are tested (see Figs 5.1 and 5.2). These 15 items cover the domains of cognition, communication, and fine and gross motor function. Each item is scored as 'typical' or 'atypical', with 'typical' implying that the defined criteria for age are met (see Chapter 5). Addition of the item scores results in the developmental scale score. The maximum score is 15 points; a score of ≤7 points is considered as atypical (Hadders-Algra et al. 2020). If an infant performs in the atypical range (score ≤7), evaluation of the infant's performance on the items belonging to a lower age column may provide an indication of the infant's degree of developmental delay.

The time needed for the developmental scale depends on the infant's age. In infants aged 2 to 3 months it takes 5 to 7 minutes; in infants aged 4 to 9 months it takes 7 to 10 minutes; and in infants aged 10 to 12 months it takes 10 to 15 minutes. These times include the recording of the scores. The scores are recorded on one of the two developmental scale assessment forms (Figs 5.1 and 5.2); one form covers the age range of 2 to 6 months (or rather the range between 6 weeks and 6.5 months), the other the age range of 7 to 12 months (or rather the range between 6.4 and 12.5 months).

The scale does not consist of 15 new items for each testing month, which would have resulted in a battery of 165 items (11 times 15 items). The developmental scale contains only 113 items as some items re-occur at multiple, adjacent ages.

Socio-Emotional Scale

The socio-emotional scale has been designed to offer professionals a tool that (1) facilitates easy, quick, and standardized assessment of the infant's socio-emotional status during the neurodevelopmental assessment; (2) is largely independent of the infant's age; and (3) to a limited extent, provides information on the infant's risk of later behavioural and emotional problems.

The scale, comprising six items, evaluates four types of behaviours: interaction, emotionality, self-regulation, and reactivity (see Chapter 6). The scores of the scale are recorded at the bottom of the assessment forms of the developmental scale (see Figs 5.1 and 5.2).

The assessment of the interaction between infant and adult (parent or assessor) is based on the age-specific cognitive and communication items of the developmental scale that are indicated on the assessment form by a red dot. If the infant scores 'typical' on at least half of the age-specific 'red dot' items, the interaction item of the socio-emotional scale is classified as typical (happy face icon), otherwise the item is classified as atypical (sad face icon).

The other five items, i.e. emotionality, self-regulation, reactivity in response to change of position, reactivity to visual stimuli, and reactivity to acoustic stimuli are scored at the end of the developmental assessment. Scoring is based on the clinical impression of the infant's behaviour during the assessment, and consists of a classification as typical (☺, happy face icon) or atypical (☹, sad face icon). The three reactivity items are used to generate a single reactivity classification, which is atypical when at least two of the three reactivity items have been scored as atypical. So (perhaps superfluously) this means that the six items of SINDA's socio-emotional scale result in a score on four types of behaviour: interaction, emotionality, self-regulation, and reactivity.

PSYCHOMETRIC PROPERTIES

The following sections describe the psychometric properties of SINDA's three scales. These properties have been evaluated in two clinical studies and in a group of infants representative of the Dutch infant population.

The two clinical studies were performed in infants who had been admitted to the Centre for Child Neurology in Frankfurt, Germany (SPZ Frankfurt-Mitte). The SPZs in Germany are specialized outpatient clinics for children at risk of or with a neurodevelopmental disorder. The SINDA scales have been implemented in the daily routines of the SPZ in Frankfurt-Mitte from 2012 onwards. Infants were included in the studies when they had been assessed with SINDA and when neurodevelopmental outcome data at the age of at least 24 months corrected age were available. The neurodevelopmental evaluation at the follow-up appointment included a standardized neurological examination and developmental testing. For the latter, the Bayley Scales of Infant Development, Second

Edition was used (Bayley 1993). The studies included 181 and 223 infants, respectively; in both studies the proportion of children diagnosed with cerebral palsy was 16%. For details of the studies see Table 3.1 and Hadders-Algra et al. 2019; Hadders-Algra 2020.

The Dutch study was designed to collect normative data for two infant assessments, i.e. the Infant Motor Profile (IMP) and the SINDA, hence its name 'IMP-SINDA project'.

Table 3.1 Characteristics of the study samples of the SPZ Frankfurt-Mitte

	Study I[a]	Study II[b]
Number of infants	181	223
Period of SINDA assessments	2012–2014	2013–2016
Sex (M/F)	92/89	117/106
Age at SINDA assessment in months CA, median (25th; 75th centiles)	3 (3; 7)	7 (3; 10)
High maternal education[c]	73/159 (46%)	87/192 (45%)
Gestational age in weeks, median (25th; 75th centiles)	30 (27; 33)	30 (28; 34)
Birthweight (g), median (25th; 75th centiles)	1305 (940; 1970)	1350 (950; 2005)
Small-for-gestational age,[d] n (%)	18 (10%)	38 (17%)
Preterm (<37 weeks gestation), n (%)	151 (83%)	180 (81%)
Brain lesions in children with a neurological diagnosis, n (%)[e]		
– IVH grade 3–4	8 (4%)	8 (3.5%)
– PVL	4 (2%)	10 (4.5%)
– Enlarged/asymmetric ventricular system	3 (2%)	6 (3%)
– Other[f]	8 (4%)	11 (5%)
Developmental outcome ≥24 months, n (%) CP	29 (16%)	35 (15.5%)
– Bilateral spastic	19 (10%)	24 (11%)
– Unilateral spastic	8 (4%)	11 (5%)
– Distribution of GMFCS level I/II/III/IV/V (n)	7/5/3/9/5	9/5/4/10/7
Other neurological diagnoses[e]	0	4 (2%)
Intellectual and/or motor disability (MDI/PDI <70)	53 (29%)	54 (24%)
Intellectual disability as single diagnosis	25 (14%)	24 (11%)
Behavioural or emotional disorder, n (%)[g]	no data available	25/165 (15%)

[a]Hadders-Algra et al. 2019. [b]Hadders-Algra et al. 2020. [c]High maternal education = university or vocational college. [d]Small for gestational age = birthweight <10th percentile. [e]Neurological diagnosis: cerebral palsy or other diagnosis, i.e. septo-optic dysplasia, Aicardie-Goutieres syndrome, CASK-mutation, and dystonia. [f]Examples of other brain lesions are pachygyria, cortical atrophy, and subdural bleeding. [g]Diagnoses according to the ICD-10, Chapter V (F). CA, corrected age; CP, cerebral palsy; GMFCS, Gross Motor Function Classification System; IVH, intraventricular haemorrhage; MDI, mental developmental index; PDI, psychomotor developmental index; PVL, periventricular leukomalacia.

Table 3.2 Characteristics of the Dutch normative sample of infants aged 2 to 12 months

Number of infants	1100
Period of SINDA assessments	2017–2019
Sex (M/F)	585/515
Age at SINDA assessment in months corrected age	100 per month of age
High maternal education, n (%)[a]	482 (44%)
Maternal non-native Dutch ethnicity, n (%)	109 (10%)
Gestational age in weeks, median (25th; 75th centiles)	39.7 (38.4; 40.7)
Birthweight (g), median (25th; 75th centiles)	3462 (3115; 3813)
Small-for-gestational age,[b] n (%)	120 (11%)
Preterm (<37 weeks gestation), n (%)	75 (6.8%)

[a]High maternal = university or vocational college. [b]Small for gestational age = birthweight <10th percentile.

The IMP is a video-based assessment of infant motor behaviour for infants aged 3 to 18 months (Heineman et al. 2011). The IMP-SINDA project included 1700 infants, aged 2 to 18 months corrected age, who were assessed with the IMP and SINDA in the period January 2017 to March 2019. The sample consisted of 100 infants for each month of age (100 2-month-olds, 100 3-month-olds, and so on up to and including 100 18-month-olds). The infants were representative of the Dutch population in terms of maternal education, ethnicity, sex, and preterm birth (see Table 3.2; Straathof et al. 2020; Wu et al. 2020). For the normative data of the SINDA only the data of the infants aged 2 to 12 months were used.

Psychometric Properties of the Neurological Scale

Two forms of reliability of the neurological scale were assessed: intrarater and interrater reliability (Hadders-Algra et al. 2019). They were determined on the basis of scores of three assessors. The reliabilities were evaluated at item level and at the level of the neurological score. The evaluation revealed that intrarater agreement on single items was substantial (Cohen's kappa-values: 0.60–0.72) and that on the neurological score was excellent (intraclass correlation coefficients [ICCs]: 0.92–0.95). The analysis of the interrater agreement resulted in similar reliability values; the agreement on single items was substantial (Cohen's kappa values: 0.57–0.67) and on the neurological score excellent (overall ICC 0.96).

In the SPZ sample the neurological score was not associated with the infant's corrected age at assessment ($\rho=-0.02$, $p=0.80$). Yet, in the general Dutch population SINDA's neurological scale showed a weak positive correlation with age at assessment ($\rho=0.28$, $p<0.001$), i.e. the neurological scores increased with increasing age at assessment. This corresponds to the clinical notion that a proportion of young infants show a

Table 3.3 Predictive values of SINDA's neurological scale

Outcome	Cerebral palsy	Atypical neurodevelopmental outcome
Sensitivity	1.00 (95% CI 0.88–1.00)	0.89 (95% CI 0.78–0.96)
	0.91 (95% CI 0.77–0.98)	0.83 (95% CI 0.72–0.91)
Specificity	0.81 (95% CI 0.74–0.87)	0.94 (95% CI 0.88–0.98)
	0.85 (95% CI 0.79–0.89)	0.96 (95% CI 0.91–0.98)

The upper data in each box are the values reported in the first study (Hadders-Algra et al. 2019), the lower data those of the second study (Hadders-Algra et al. 2020). CI, confidence interval.

transient neurological impairment that usually resolves in the second half of the first year (Michaelis et al. 1993; Nuysink et al. 2013).

The sensitivity and specificity of an 'at risk' neurological score (≤21) were calculated in both clinical studies, not only in terms of prediction of cerebral palsy but also in terms of prediction of any atypical neurodevelopmental outcome. The latter was defined as the presence of a clear neurological syndrome such as cerebral palsy or the presence of a mental and/or psychomotor developmental index of <70. The data are summarized in Table 3.3. They indicate that SINDA's neurological scale has satisfactory predictive properties in the setting of the SPZ.

Psychometric Properties of the Developmental Scale

Interrater reliability of the developmental scale was determined in 60 consecutively recruited infants aged 6 weeks to 12 months corrected age assessed in the IMP-SINDA project during the autumn of 2018. Each infant was assessed by two assessors from a pool of six people; the combinations of the two people assessing a single infant varied. The correlation between the developmental scores of the pairs of assessors was consistently high, with an overall correlation of the scores of the 60 infants of ρ=0.97 (p<0.001).

In the SPZ-population the infant's developmental score showed a negative correlation with age at assessment (ρ=−0.33, p<0.001), implying that the developmental scores decreased with increasing age at assessment. However, inspection of the data suggested that this correlation was largely brought about by the referral pattern to the SPZ: infants referred at the age of 6 months corrected age or older had significantly more often an atypical outcome than the infants who were referred before the age of 6 months. When the evaluation of the association between developmental score and age at assessment was repeated for the two age groups separately, the association with age disappeared (infants <6 months: ρ=−0.04, p=0.69; infants ≥6 months: ρ=−0.012, p=0.896; Hadders-Algra et al. 2020). In the general Dutch population,

SINDA's developmental scale showed a weak negative correlation with age at assessment ($\rho=-0.13$, $p<0.001$). The low value of the correlation coefficient indicates that this association has limited clinical value.

In the SPZ population an atypical developmental score (≤7 points) predicted intellectual disability well, i.e. with a sensitivity of 0.77 and a specificity of 0.92. Information of the developmental score in children with a typical neurological score did not improve prediction of atypical outcome. However, in children with an atypical neurological score, addition of the information of the developmental score improved prediction of atypical neurodevelopmental outcome (Hadders-Algra et al. 2020).

Psychometric Properties of the Socio-Emotional Scale

Interrater reliability of the socio-emotional scale was determined on the basis of the same 60 infants of the IMP-SINDA project with the same team of assessors as the interrater reliability of the developmental scale. The agreement between the pairs of assessors on the four behaviours of the socio-emotional scale was excellent (Cohen's kappa values: 0.78–0.90).

In the SPZ study no association between the infant's age at assessment and socio-emotional behaviour scores were found for three of the four behaviours: emotionality: $r=-0.02$, $p=0.84$; self-regulation: $r=-0.15$, $p=0.05$; reactivity: $r=0.03$, $p=0.74$. Interaction, which depends on performance on the developmental scale, was (like the developmental scale itself) correlated with age ($r=-0.34$, $p<0.001$). However, when the bias induced by the referral pattern was taken into account and the associations between interaction and infant age at assessment were assessed in the two age subgroups, the correlation between interaction and age largely disappeared (infants <6 months: $\rho=0.05$, $p=0.69$; infants ≥6 months: $r=-0.20$, $p=0.06$; Hadders-Algra et al. 2020). In the general Dutch population emotionality and self-regulation were also not associated with the infant's age ($r=0.01$, $p=0.83$ and $r=0.01$, $p=0.78$, respectively). Yet, reactivity showed a weak positive correlation with age ($r=0.12$, $p<0.001$) and interaction showed a weak negative correlation ($r=-0.28$, $p<0.001$). The correlation coefficient of the former association was low, indicating that this association had limited clinical value. Yet, the negative correlation between age and interaction may reflect an effect of the stranger's anxiety that may emerge in the second half of the first year (Super and Harkness 2015). The SPZ study indicated that atypical emotionality and atypical self-regulation during infancy were associated with the presence of a behavioural or emotional disorder at the age of at least 2 years. The specificity of both infant behaviours to predict a later behavioural or emotional disorder was high (0.85 and 0.98, respectively), but their sensitivity was relatively low (0.32 and 0.40, respectively). Our data indicated in general that, on the one hand, infants who show atypical emotionality or atypical self-regulation had a high risk to be later diagnosed with a behavioural or emotional disorder. On the other hand, the absence of atypical emotionality or atypical self-regulation did not preclude the development of a behavioural or emotional disorder. These findings correspond to the moderate associations between infant temperament and attachment and later behavioural outcome reported in the literature. These associations reflect the multifactorial origin of behavioural disorders (Bohlin and Hagekull 2009).

Atypical SINDA scores on interaction and reactivity were not associated with behavioural outcome at 2 years (Hadders-Algra et al. 2020).

IMPLEMENTATION OF SINDA IN CLINICAL PRACTICE

In this section we discuss the practicalities of SINDA. They address (1) the importance of the infant's behavioural state; (2) the role of the parents; and (3) the conditions during the assessment.

Behavioural State

The behavioural state of the infant has a large impact on the results of a neurodevelopmental examination (Prechtl 1977). For instance, crying induces a reduction in movement variation and promotes stereotypies (Hadders-Algra 2004), and drowsiness interferes with tasks requiring attention. This means that an adequate behavioural state is a prerequisite for the performance of SINDA: the infant needs to be awake and as alert as possible, and should not be fussy or crying.

The order in which the assessment is carried out is largely governed by the infant's behavioural state. In infants with a 'fragile' behavioural state it is recommended to start with items that can be performed while the infant sits on the parent's lap. In other children, the assessment usually starts with the assessment of spontaneous movements, either on an assessment couch or on a mattress on the floor. The best way to facilitate an adequate behavioural state in the infant is to conduct the assessment in the style of play.

During SINDA the assessor continuously monitors the infant's behavioural state; it is recorded on each assessment form. If the infant does not meet the criteria of an adequate behavioural state, the following strategies may be followed: (1) temporarily interrupt the assessment, e.g. to feed a hungry and crying infant; (2) make a new appointment for the assessment; and (3) continue with the assessment while acknowledging that the results of the assessment have limited value.

Parents

Parents are the key people in the infant's life. They provide the health professional performing SINDA with essential information on the child's history and the infant's behaviour and achievements in daily life. The relevant information is recorded at the top of the assessment form of the neurological scale.

During SINDA the parents are present, and during parts of the assessment the infant sits on a parent's lap. After the completion of SINDA the parents are informed about the results and the significance of the findings of the assessment (see Chapter 7).

Conditions During the Assessment

SINDA can be performed in any environment that ensures that the infant is in an adequate behavioural state. This also means that the environment should contain as few distractors as possible. This may, for instance, mean that parents are reminded to take care that an accompanying sibling does not interfere with the assessment.

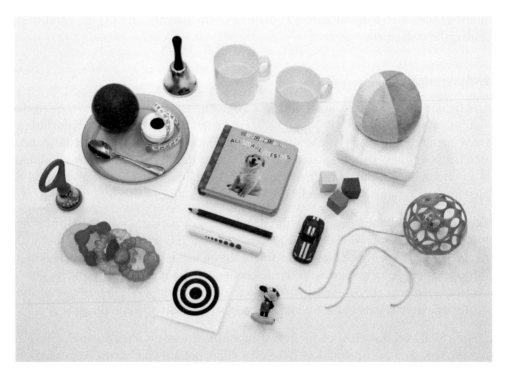

Figure 3.1 Example of the testing material used in SINDA

The material needed for the neurological and developmental scales partially overlap. For both scales attractive toys are needed to engage the infant in movement and play activities: relatively small rings, puppets (infants love Mickey Mouse figures!), balls, and cars. Additionally, the neurological scale requests a penlight (or the light from a smartphone) and a measurement tape. A retractable measurement tape that flips back into its case not only serves the measurement of the infant's head circumference, but it is also an excellent means to test whether an infant is able to generate a pincer grasp (a developmental item at 12 months). Specific objects needed for the developmental scale are a bull's eye (which you can easily make yourself), a plate, a spoon, two cups, a picture book, a pencil, a bell, balls, some cubes, a cloth, a ball or ring on a string, and an additional identical string.

A requirement of the assessment room is that it allows for infant play behaviour. This implies that (1) the floor is compatible with infant creeping and crawling; (2) it has a mattress to lie or sit on; and (3) it contains furniture that the infant may use to pull themself into standing position, such as a sofa, a small chair, or a stool. In addition, the room needs to have chairs for the parents and the assessor, and a table that is placed in such a way that parent and infant can sit opposite the assessor.

SINDA requires a set of toys and objects that can be easily purchased in toy shops and/or on the Internet (Fig. 3.1). In other words, SINDA does not require an expensive assessment tool kit.

INTRODUCTION TO THE CHAPTERS WITH THE DESCRIPTION OF THE ITEMS

The following three chapters contain the descriptions of the SINDA items: Chapter 4 covers the neurological scale, Chapter 5 the developmental scale, and Chapter 6 the socio-emotional scale. The items are illustrated with figures and videos. The videos are available online (see access details on page xi).

In Chapter 7 (Tables 7.1–7.3), the prevalence of atypical performance in the Dutch normative population are provided. The data confirm that the items vary in difficulty, which underlines the proper construct of SINDA.

## CHAPTER 4

The Neurological Scale

INTRODUCTION AND GENERAL PRINCIPLES

The Standardized Infant NeuroDevelopmental Assessment (SINDA) neurological scale is a concise neurological assessment of infants aged 6 weeks to 12 months corrected age. It has five domains assessing spontaneous movements (eight items), cranial nerve function (seven items), motor reactions to postural stimulation (five items), muscle tone (four items), and reflexes and reactions (four items). Each item is scored as 'typical' or 'atypical' according to the criteria described in this chapter.

In many items the presence of stereotypy and/or asymmetry results in the assignment of 'atypical'. To this end we use the following criteria:

- A *stereotypy* means that a specific posture or movement pattern dominates the assessment, and other postures and movements occur only occasionally. Dominant stereotypies result in the classification 'atypical'.

- An *asymmetry* in movements and postures is scored as 'atypical' when the infant shows a consistent asymmetry. This implies that asymmetries that can be observed occasionally are not classified as 'atypical'. In the case of a consistent asymmetry, the side that performs atypically is recorded (on the right side of the assessment form). Note that in the case of a consistent asymmetry, it is not always evident which side is the atypical or most affected side. For instance, in the case of atypical stretch reflexes, it may be difficult to determine whether the side that responds more strongly or the one that responds more weakly is the atypical side. We suggest recording the asymmetry as accurately as possible.

In the case of atypical performance, the type of atypical behaviour is recorded on the assessment form by underlining or circling the atypical behaviour that has been observed. If the assessor is in doubt whether the infant's performance on a specific item is typical or atypical, the behaviour is classified as 'typical' ('benefit of the doubt principle').

Note that SINDA is not based on video recording. This means that the scoring of asymmetries and stereotypies is based on the gestalt during the clinical assessment.

Behavioural State, the Order of the Assessment, and Head Position

Figure 4.1 displays the assessment form of the neurological scale. An adequate behavioural state is a prerequisite for the assessment (see Chapter 3). This means that the infant should be awake, alert, and moving most of the time. The infant should not be assessed while crying or sleeping. The behavioural state is recorded on the assessment form by ticking one of the boxes at the top of the form: wakeful, alert/sleepy, tired/fussy/crying (which precludes proper assessment) and sub-acute illness, e.g. infection, post-operative condition. The behaviour that represents the overall behavioural state best is recorded.

In general, the assessment starts with the observation of spontaneous movements. In young infants the assessment usually starts in supine, in older infants in the sitting position. Spontaneous movements are observed for 3 to 5 minutes. Next, cranial nerve functions are assessed, and thereafter the other item sections follow. The actual order of assessment is not very important; the sequence mentioned in the manual is a convenient one and also one that is associated with a high chance of the maintenance of an adequate behavioural state in the infant. Some items are based on observation (indicated with an O on the left side of the assessment form), others on specific testing, i.e. actions performed by the assessor (indicated with T on the assessment form). Videos 4.1 and 4.2 illustrate an assessment in an infant aged 5 and 9 months, respectively.

The positions in which the items may be assessed most easily are indicated on the left-hand side of the assessment form. The following abbreviations are used:
- A = all: the item may be tested or observed in any position
- P = prone
- PS = prone suspension
- Si = sitting (with or without support)
- SS = supine suspension
- Su = supine
- VS = vertical suspension

Some infants have a clear head turn preference to one side. If that happens, care should be taken to assess muscle tone and reflexes with the head in the midline position, as the head preference position may induce asymmetries in muscle tone and reflexes. We suggest using one of the following two assessment strategies. The first strategy is to position the infant's head in the midline, for instance with the help of a small support pillow in the infant lying supine. Next, the infant's muscle tone and reflexes are assessed with the head in the midline position. The second strategy consists of first assessing muscle tone and reflexes with the head turned to the infant's preferred side. Next, the

SINDA Neurological scale

Behavioural state	☐ awake, alert	☐ sleepy, tired	
	☐ fussy	☐ crying	☐ sub-acute illness
Paroxysmal events	☐ absent	☐ suspect	☐ obvious
Head	☐ ....cm	☐ macrocephaly	☐ microcephaly
	☐ plagiocephaly	☐ atypical fontanelle	☐ atypical sutures
Additional	☐ somatic symptoms	☐ sev. vis. impairment	☐ dysmorphic signs
		☐ sev. aud. impairment	☐ atypical phonation

Name:..

Birth date:.................................... ♂ / ♀

Corr. Age:...

Date:..

Examiner:...

Hospital:..

Additional clinical comments:...

Pos *	O,T#	item	typical (1)	atypical (0)	worst side	score
A1 Spontaneous movements (local)						
1 A	O	Head & neck & trunk	varied & symmetric	stereotyped posture, opisthotonus, asymmetric	R L	
2 A	O	Arms	varied & symmetric	stereotyped posture, asymmetric	R L	
3 A	O	Hands	varied & symmetric	stereotyped posture, asymmetric	R L	
4 A	O	Legs	varied & symmetric	stereotyped posture, asymmetric	R L	
5 A	O	Feet	varied & symmetric	stereotyped posture, asymmetric	R L	
6 Su	O	ATNR	absent, occasionally present	frequently, continuously present, asymmetric		
A2 Spontaneous movements (general)						
7 A	O	Quality	varied & symmetric & fluent & isolated movements of fingers & toes	stereotyped, jerky, jittery, startles, tremulous, sluggish, stiff, no isolated movements of fingers, toes, asymmetric	R L	
8 A	O	Quantity	moderate & changing over time	predominantly hypokinetic, predominantly hyperkinetic		
B Cranial nerves						
9 A	O	Facial appearance	varied & symmetric	expressionless, asymmetric	R L	
10 A	O	Oral motor behaviour	mouth mostly closed & tongue within the mouth & no obvious drooling	mouth mostly open, stereotyped tongue protrusion, fasciculations, obvious drooling		
11 Su, Si	T	Glabella reflex	moderate threshold & moderate intensity & symmetric	low, high threshold, low, high intensity, asymmetric		
12 Su, Si	O T	Eye position & eye movements	fixates & parallel position & conjugated movements	no fixation, predominant strabismus, unconjugated movements, restricted motility, sunset, nystagmus	R L	
13 Su, Si	T	Optical blink reflex	blinks & symmetric	absent, doubtful, delayed, asymmetric	R L	
14 Su, Si	T	Pupillary reaction	direct & indirect: prompt & symmetric	absent, slow, tonic, asymmetric	R L	
15 Su, Si	T	Acoustic reaction to clapping	blinks, facial reaction	absent, doubtful		
C Motor reactions to postural stimulation						
16 Su	T	Pull-to-sit	activation of neck & shoulder & arm muscles & symmetric arm activity & adequate flexion hips	head lag, active retroflexion, no or minimal muscle activation, asymmetric, inadequate hip flexion	R L	
17 P	O	Head in prone	lifts head as selective action	does not lift head, stereotyped hyperextension		
18 PS	T	Prone suspension	head in line, above trunk level	head, trunk floppy, stereotyped, opisthotonus		
19 VS	T	Vertical suspension	head upright & appropriate axillary resistance & legs varied & symmetric	poor head control, slipping through, stereotyped leg movements, asymmetric	R L	
20 VS	T	Feet touching the ground	varied feet postures & movements & symmetric	stereotyped feet postures, asymmetric	R L	
D Muscle tone						
21 Su, SS	T	Tone of neck & trunk	moderate resistance against passive movements	consistent hypotonia, consistent hypertonia, sudden changes in muscle tone		
22 Su, Si	T	Resistance against passive movements, arm traction	symmetric & moderate resistance against passive movements & slight elbow flexion	consistent hypotonia, consistent hypertonia, sudden changes in muscle tone, asymmetric	R L	
23 Su, Si	T	Resistance against passive movements, leg traction	symmetric & moderate resistance against passive movements & slight knee flexion	consistent hypotonia, consistent hypertonia, sudden changes in muscle tone, asymmetric	R L	
24 Su, Si	T	Feet: resistance against passive movements	symmetric & moderate resistance against passive movements	consistent hypotonia, consistent hypertonia, sudden changes in muscle tone, ankle clonus, positive catch phenomenon, asymmetric	R L	
E Reflexes and reactions						
25 Su, Si	T	Upper extremities: biceps reflex	symmetric positive response	areflexia, asymmetric	R L	
26 Su, Si	T	Lower extremities: knee jerk & ankle clone	symmetric positive response	areflexia, tonic response, clonus, asymmetric	R L	
27 Su, Si	T	Foot sole sensibility	withdrawal of legs & varied toe movement & symmetric	no reaction, stereotyped toe movements, asymmetric	R L	
28 Su, Si	T	Foot sole response	varied dorsiflexion 1st toe & toe spreading & symmetric	stereotyped, tonic dorsi- or plantar flexion, no or weak response, asymmetric	R L	
				SINDA Neurological Score		

* Pos: Position; A: All; P: Prone; PS: Prone Suspension; S: (supported) Sitting; Su: Supine; SS: Supine Suspension; VS: Vertical Suspension.
# O: Observational item; T: Test item.
ATNR, asymmetrical tonic neck response.

© M. Hadders-Algra, U. Tacke,
H. Philippi & J. Pietz
Oct 2021

Figure 4.1 SINDA neurological scale assessment form Typical performance is credited with 1 point, atypical performance with a 0. The type of atypical performance is recorded by underlining the type of atypical behaviour in the 'atypical' column. Asymmetries are recorded by circling the worst side. Addition of the number of points results in SINDA's neurological score that is recorded at the bottom of the form. A score of ≤21 points indicates an 'at risk' score, implying that the infant is at increased risk of a neurodevelopmental disorder. Additional clinical details, including the infant's behavioural state, are recorded at the top of the form. A digital version of the form is available online (see access details on page xi).

assessor turns the infant's head to the contralateral side and repeats the assessment of muscle tone and reflexes with the head in this position. In general, the first strategy is more successful than the second.

General Remarks on the Assessment Form

At the top of the assessment form also information on paroxysmal events, on the head, including its circumference and the presence of an atypical form, and additional physical impairments are recorded. This information is not used to calculate SINDA's neurological score, but it facilitates the interpretation of the infant's neurological performance.

The & sign on the assessment form denotes that the criteria that are connected by the & sign both need to be fulfilled; a comma between options denotes alternatives, not obligatory combinations.

PAROXYSMAL EVENTS

Paroxysmal events occurring during the assessment are recorded as follows:

- absent, i.e. no seizure activity observed;
- suspect: behaviour may imply the presence of paroxysmal events, seizure activity;
- obvious: behaviour is without doubt expression of paroxysmal events indicating seizure activity or evident seizure activity.

Signs that may reflect seizure activity are staring, loss of consciousness, apnoea, stereo-typed eye movements, stiffening of the body, or clonic movements (Alam and Lux 2012).

HEAD

Head circumference should be measured and recorded. In general, infants are not fond of the measurement of head circumference. The measurement is therefore best performed at the end of the assessment. It is recommended to assess head circumference while the infant is either held in the parent's arms or sitting on the parent's lap. A trick that often works is to offer the infant the measurement tape and let them play with the tape (which also allows for the evaluation of manual skills and the quality of upper extremity movements); next, the infant holds on to the end of the tape, while the assessor quickly puts the tape's beginning around the infant's head (Fig. 4.2). The tape (retractable or not) has to be a non-stretchable 'lasso' tape, which measures in centimetres with one decimal number. The head circumference, i.e. the occipitofrontal circumference, is the largest circumference that can be measured. Head circumference is measured twice, of which the largest measure is recorded with one decimal.

The assessment of the head also includes the assessment of the fontanelle, in particular the large fontanelle, and the palpation of the sutures. In addition, the form of the head is noted.

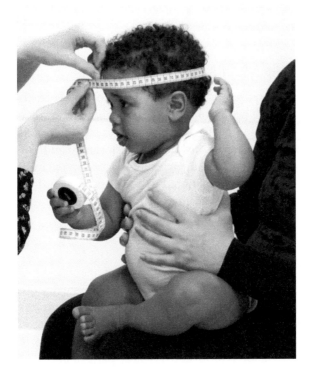

Figure 4.2 Measurement of head circumference

The information on the head is recorded as follows:

- head circumference: in decimal centimetres;
- macrocephaly, i.e. head circumference ≥97 percentile;
- microcephaly, i.e. head circumference ≤3rd percentile;
- plagiocephaly: this box is ticked when the infant shows a positional plagiocephaly (an asymmetrical distortion of the skull) or other marked deformities of the skull, such as deformities due to premature fusion of cranial sutures (e.g. scaphocephaly, a long and narrow head due to premature fusion of the sagittal suture; brachicephaly, a broad and short head, due to coronal craniosynostosis; turricephaly, i.e. brachicephaly in combination with an increased height in the cephalocaudal dimension of the head). The type of deformity is recorded;
- atypical fontanelle, e.g. tense or bulging fontanelle, sunken fontanelle;
- atypical sutures, e.g. overlapping bones or widened sutures.

ADDITIONAL INFORMATION ON PHYSICAL IMPAIRMENTS

Finally, the presence of significant somatic symptoms (e.g. hepatosplenomegaly), clinically clear forms of severe visual and hearing impairment, dysmorphic signs, and atypical phonation (e.g. weak or high pitched) are recorded, as this information may affect the interpretation of the neurological findings.

Interpretation of the Results

Addition of the item scores results in SINDA's neurological score. The maximum score is 28 points. A score of ≤21 points indicates that the infant is at risk of a neurodevelopmental disorder (Hadders-Algra et al. 2019). The presence of an 'at risk' score indicates the need for careful monitoring of the infant's development and/or further diagnostics and the need for early intervention. The neurological assessment by itself does not result in a specific diagnosis. It should be noted that the assessment does not allow for the detection of unilateral hearing impairment. Further details on the interpretation of the neurological findings are discussed in Chapter 7.

Description of the Items

In the following sections the items of the neurological scale are described. The description of each item starts with the item's name and whether the item is based on observation (indicated by an O) or on a specific testing procedure (indicated by a T). Next, the description continues with information on the assessment method, the preferred testing position, and the criteria for 'typical' and 'atypical' performance.

Note that in the description of typical performance the word 'and' (or on the assessment form the sign '&') means that all criteria connected by the 'and' (&) need to be met in order to be scored as typical.

'SPONTANEOUS MOVEMENTS' DOMAIN

The eight items on spontaneous movements (local and general) are only assessed during the periods in which the infant is allowed to produce self-generated movements. This means that the behaviour of the infant while the assessor touches the infant are not taken into account.

The self-generated movements are observed throughout the assessment, but at the beginning of the assessment a period of at least 3 minutes is dedicated to spontaneous movements. Depending on the infant's age and abilities, the spontaneous movements are observed in any position, i.e. in supine, prone, sitting, standing, and walking. In young infants, in whom the assessment usually starts in supine, the behaviour in supine position contributes substantially to the gestalt of the quality of spontaneous movements. Nevertheless, in young infants spontaneous movements in other positions, e.g. in prone position, are also taken into account. This also implies that the items of the spontaneous movements domain are recorded at the end of the assessment.

The first six items assess the movements of a specific part of the body (spontaneous movements, local), the following two items address spontaneous movements in the entire body (spontaneous movements, general).

Item 1 Head & Neck & Trunk: Movements and Postures (0)

Position

This item is assessed in all positions used. This is indicated on the assessment form with an A for all positions.

Procedure

The spontaneous movements and postures of the head, neck, and trunk are observed throughout the assessment.

Scoring

1 = typical   Varied and symmetric (Fig. 4.3).
0 = atypical   Presence of at least one of the following signs:
                    - stereotyped posture
                    - opisthotonus
                    - asymmetric: an asymmetric head position is present when the infant has a head preference to one side and is not able to turn the head (to a considerable extent) to the other side. Another criterion for asymmetry is the presence of a clear convexity in the trunk only present on one side of the body (Fig. 4.4). Record atypical side, i.e. the non-preferred side of the head, and the most convex side of the trunk: R/L.

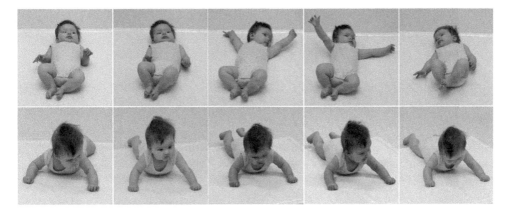

Figure 4.3 Varied and symmetric movements and postures of head, neck, and trunk in an infant aged 4 months (Item 1) The variants are more clearly expressed in supine than in prone.

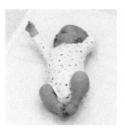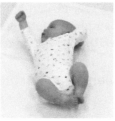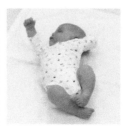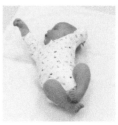

Figure 4.4 Atypical movements and postures of head, neck, and trunk in an infant aged 3 months (Item 1) Stereotyped hyperextension of neck and trunk with head preference posture to the right side.

Item 2 Arms: Movements and Postures (0)

POSITION

This item is assessed in all positions used. This is indicated on the assessment form with an A for all positions.

PROCEDURE

The spontaneous movements and postures of the arms are observed throughout the assessment.

SCORING

1 = typical   Varied and symmetric (Fig. 4.5 and Video 4.3).
0 = atypical   Presence of at least one of the following signs:
                 - stereotyped posture, i.e. specific posture strikingly often present, such as elbow flexion, elbow extension, lower arm pronation. Stereotypy means that the posture or movement dominates the assessment and other postures and movements occur only occasionally (Fig. 4.6 and Video 4.4)
                 - asymmetric, record atypical side: R/L.

Item 3 Hands: Movements and Postures (0)

POSITION

This item is assessed in all positions used. This is indicated on the assessment form with an A for all positions.

PROCEDURE

The spontaneous movements and postures of the hands, including the wrists and fingers, are observed throughout the assessment.

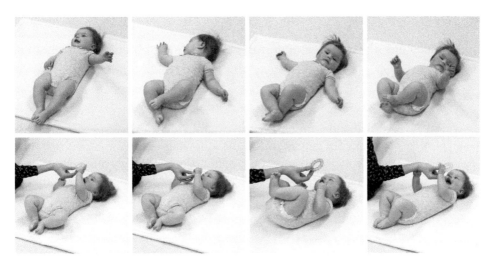

Figure 4.5 Varied and symmetric movements and postures of the arms and hands in an infant aged 6 months (Items 2 and 3)

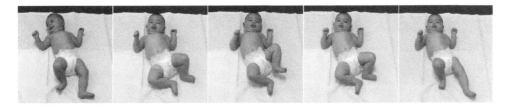

Figure 4.6 Atypical movements and postures of the arms and hands in an infant aged 4 months (Items 2 and 3) The infant shows reduced variation in the movements of arms and hands; the arms are mainly flexed and the hands in fists.

SCORING

1 = typical	Varied and symmetric (Fig. 4.5 and Video 4.3).
0 = atypical	Presence of at least one of the following signs:

- stereotyped posture, i.e. specific posture strikingly often present, such as fisting. Stereotypy means that the posture or movement dominates the assessment and other postures and movements occur only occasionally (Fig. 4.6 and Video 4.4)
- asymmetric, record atypical side: R/L.

Item 4 Legs: Movements and Postures (0)

POSITION

This item is assessed in all positions used. This is indicated on the assessment form with an A for all positions.

Procedure

The spontaneous movements and postures of the legs are observed throughout the assessment.

Scoring

1 = typical	Varied and symmetric (Fig. 4.7 and Video 4.5)
0 = atypical	Presence of at least one of the following signs:

- stereotyped posture, i.e. specific posture strikingly often present, such as such as leg extension, feet tiptoeing. Stereotypy means that the posture or movement dominates the assessment, and other postures and movements occur only occasionally (Fig. 4.8 and Video 4.6)
- asymmetric, record atypical side: R/L.

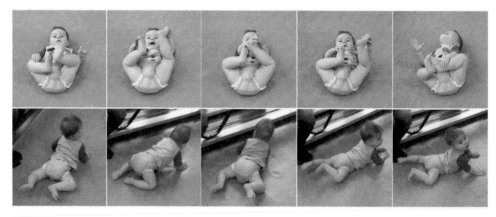

Figure 4.7 Varied and symmetric movements and postures of the legs and feet in an infant aged 10 months (Items 4 and 5)

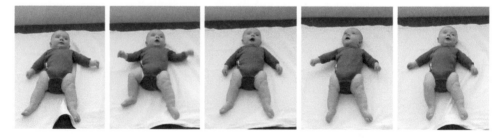

Figure 4.8 Atypical movements and postures of the legs and feet in an infant aged 4 months (Items 4 and 5)

Item 5 Feet: Movements and Postures (0)

POSITION

This item is assessed in all positions used. This is indicated on the assessment form with an A for all positions.

PROCEDURE

The spontaneous movements and postures of the feet, including the ankles and toes, are observed throughout the assessment.

SCORING

1 = typical	Varied and symmetric (Fig. 4.7 and Video 4.5).
0 = atypical	Presence of at least one of the following signs:

- stereotyped posture, i.e. specific posture strikingly often present, such as clawing, dorsiflexion of the first toe. Stereotypy means that the posture or movement dominates the assessment, and other postures and movements occur only occasionally (Fig. 4.8 and Video 4.6)
- asymmetric, record atypical side: R/L.

Item 6 Asymmetrical Tonic Neck Response (ATNR) (0)

The ATNR implies that the head position induces reflex posturing of the limbs. More specifically, a sideward rotation of the head results in an increase of the tone of the extensor muscles of the limbs on the facial side of the body and in a decrease of extensor tone on the contralateral side. In other words, the ATNR induces a 'fencing posture' in which the arm on the side to which the face is turned extends and the contralateral flexes at the elbow (Magnus and de Kleijn 1912; Peiper 1963). A corresponding posturing in the legs may also be observed. ATNR activity is present at all ages, including typical adults (Bruijn et al. 2013). However, typical brain function easily overrules ATNR activity, allowing individuals with typical brain function to move their limbs independently of head position. The same holds true for infants: typically developing infants infrequently show ATNR postures. The presence of frequent or obligatory, i.e. stereotyped, ATNR posturing indicates the presence of brain dysfunction (Peiper 1963).

POSITION

The ATNR is best observed during spontaneous movements in supine (Su).

PROCEDURE

The *spontaneous* occurrence of the ATNR during the assessment is noted. As noted above, the ATNR pattern consists of extension of the limbs on the 'facial' side of the body and flexion of the limbs on the 'occipital' side. In general, the pattern is more clearly present

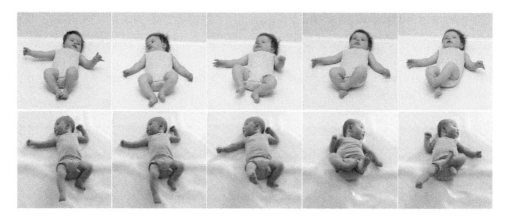

Figure 4.9 ATNR: typical and atypical performance (Item 6) Upper panel: typical perfor-mance with an occasionally occurring asymmetrical tonic neck response (ATNR). In the third frame the infant shows the ATNR pattern in the arms: extension of the arm on the facial side and a tendency to flex the arm on the occipital side. The legs do not participate in the ATNR-patterning. Lower panel: atypical performance with frequently occurring ATNR.

in the upper limbs than in the lower limbs and may be less clearly expressed on the 'occipital' side of the body.

SCORING

1 = typical	ATNR absent or occasionally present (Fig. 4.9).
0 = atypical	Presence of at least one of the following signs:
	- frequently or continuously present
	- asymmetric, record atypical side: R/L.

Item 7 Quality of Spontaneous Movements in General (0)

POSITION

This item is assessed in all positions used. This is indicated on the assessment form with an A for all positions.

PROCEDURE

The quality of spontaneous movements of all parts of the body is observed throughout the assessment.

SCORING

1 = typical   Varied and symmetric and fluent (Video 4.7). A high frequency (>6Hz), small amplitude (<3cm) tremor during crying may be present (Prechtl 1977).

0 = atypical   Presence of at least one of the following signs:
- stereotyped (Video 4.8)
- 'startles', jerky, jittery motility
- stiff motility
- frequently occurring tremors
- sluggish
- no isolated movements of fingers, toes
- asymmetric, record atypical side: R/L.

Item 8 Quantity of Spontaneous Movements in General   (0)

POSITION

This item is assessed in all positions used. This is indicated on the assessment form with an A for all positions.

PROCEDURE

The quantity of spontaneous movements is observed throughout the assessment.

SCORING

1 = typical   Moderate quantity and quantity changes over time (Video 4.7; the infant on this video does not only show movements with a typical quality but also with a typical quantity).
Note: quantity may be typical in the presence of repetitive, stereotyped movements, i.e. movements with an atypical quality.

0 = atypical   Presence of at least one of the following signs:
- predominantly hypokinetic; the assessor has the impression that when movements would have been filmed on video, velocity of replay has been slowed down by a factor of two (Video 4.9)
- predominantly hyperkinetic; the assessor has the impression that when movements would have been filmed on video, velocity of replay has been sped up by a factor of two (Video 4.10).

'CRANIAL NERVES' DOMAIN

Item 9 Facial Appearance   (0)

POSITION

This item is assessed in all positions used. This is indicated on the assessment form with an A for all positions.

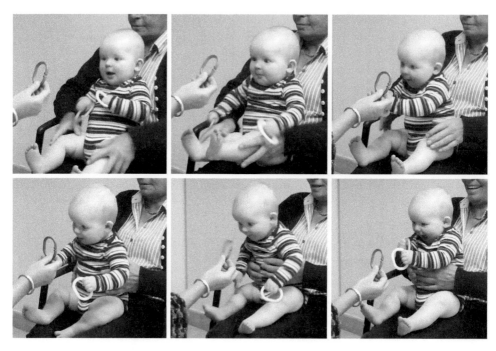

Figure 4.10 Varied and symmetric facial expressions in an infant aged 4 months (Item 9)

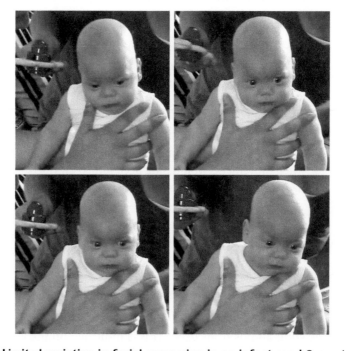

Figure 4.11 Limited variation in facial expression in an infant aged 3 months (Item 9)

PROCEDURE

Facial movements and expressions are observed throughout the assessment.

SCORING

1 = typical	Varied and symmetric facial movements and expressions (Fig. 4.10 and Video 4.11). Note: some asymmetry may be observed, in particular during crying.
0 = atypical	Presence of at least one of the following signs: - expressionless, limited variation in facial expression (Fig. 4.11) - predominantly asymmetric, record atypical side: R/L.

Item 10 Oral Motor Behaviour (0)

POSITION

This item is assessed in all positions used. This is indicated on the assessment form with an A for all positions.

PROCEDURE

Behaviour of the mouth and tongue, and the presence of drooling are observed throughout the assessment.

SCORING

1 = typical	Mouth mostly closed and tongue within mouth and no obvious drooling.
0 = atypical	Presence of at least one of the following signs: - mouth most of the time open (Fig. 4.12) - stereotyped tongue protrusion (Fig. 4.13) - tongue fasciculation - obvious drooling.

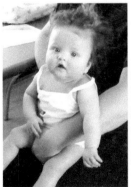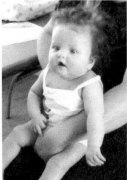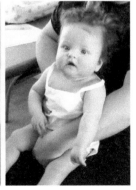

Figure 4.12 **Atypical oral motor behaviour (Item 10): mouth mostly open**

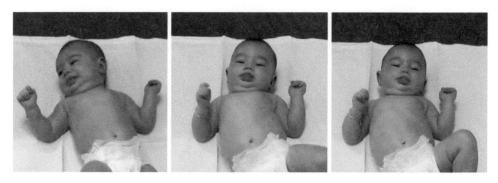

Figure 4.13 Atypical oral motor behaviour (Item 10): stereotyped tongue protrusion

Item 11 Glabella Reflex (T)

POSITION

The glabella reflex is best assessed in supine (Su) or sitting (Si).

PROCEDURE

Tap briskly on the glabella, i.e. the skin between the eyebrows and above the nose (Fig. 4.14). Perform the tap two to three times with an interval of about 2 seconds. Evaluate the threshold, i.e. the ease with which the response may be elicited, and the response intensity and symmetry.

SCORING

1 = typical   Symmetric, quick closure of the eyes and moderate response threshold and response intensity (Video 4.12).

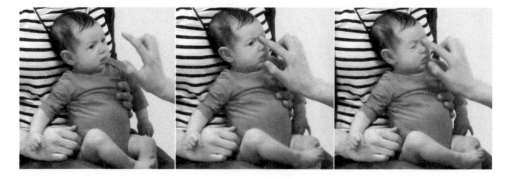

Figure 4.14 Assessment of the glabella reflex (Item 11)

0 = atypical   Presence of at least one of the following signs:
- no or minimal response
- low threshold and/or high intensity: the response is easily elicited, i.e. with a weak tap, and results in accompanying movements of the head (Video 4.13)
- asymmetric, record atypical side: R/L.

Item 12 Position and Movements of the Eyes   (O&T)

Position

The position and movements of the eyes are best assessed in supine (Su) or sitting (Si).

Procedure

The position and movements of the eyes are observed throughout the assessment. In addition, eye movements are assessed during visual pursuit of an attractive object, e.g. a small Mickey Mouse puppet. In young infants a bull's eye may also be used (Figs 4.15 and 4.16). While the infant is lying supine or sitting on the parent's lap the object is moved at a distance of 20cm to 30cm, starting in the midline and moving laterally to right and left, next moving vertically and obliquely towards the nose (Video 4.14).

Scoring

1 = typical   Fixates (briefly or for a longer period), parallel position of the eyes and conjugated eye movements. Alternating convergent strabismus may occur occasionally.

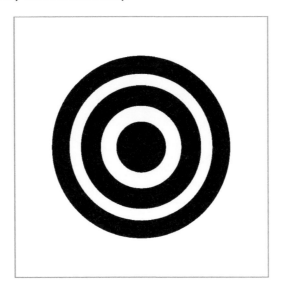

Figure 4.15 Bull's eye

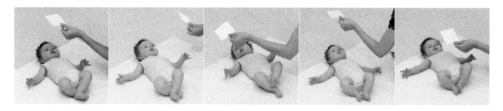

Figure 4.16 Assessment position and movements of the eyes (Item 12) The assessor uses a bull's eye to test position and movements of the eyes in an infant aged 4 months. The assessment starts with central fixation, next the assessor tests eye movements to the left, to the right, upwards, and downwards.

0 = atypical   Presence of at least one of the following signs (Fig. 4.17):
- does not show any sign of visual fixation
- divergent strabismus
- vertical strabismus

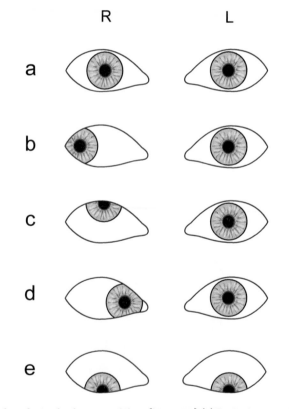

Figure 4.17 Typical and atypical eye position (Item 12) (a) Typical, centred, and symmetrical eye position; (b) divergent strabism right eye; (c) vertical strabism right eye; (d) convergent strabism right eye; (e) sunset phenomenon (both eyes).

- frequently occurring bilateral convergent strabismus (Video 4.15)
- unilateral strabismus that is not consistently present while the other eye has a normal position
- unconjugated eye movements
- restricted motility in any direction, e.g. due to abducens paresis or vertical gaze paresis
- sunset (eyes tend to point downwards; as a result the eyes mostly show white sclera in combination with partially downwardly disappearing irises, giving the impression of 'sunset')
- nystagmus.

Item 13 Optical Blink   (T)

POSITION

The optical blink is best assessed in supine (Su) or sitting (Si).

PROCEDURE

Shine sudden flashlight at one or both eyes. Care should be taken that the environmental light conditions are not too bright.

SCORING

1 = typical	Fast and symmetrical blinking of the eyes (Video 4.16). In most typically developing infants the blink reaction habituates after a few trials.
0 = atypical	Presence of at least one of the following signs: - absent or doubtful or delayed response - asymmetric, record atypical side: R/L.

Item 14 Pupillary Reaction   (T)

POSITION

The pupillary reaction is best assessed in supine (Su) or sitting (Si).

PROCEDURE

The size of the pupil is observed. Then a bright light is flashed into one eye only and the reactions of both pupils observed. The easiest way to prevent a direct light stimulus in the contralateral eye is to put the examiner's hand as a barrier between the eyes (Fig. 4.18 and Video 4.17). The procedure is repeated with the other eye. Care should be taken that the environmental light conditions are not too bright.

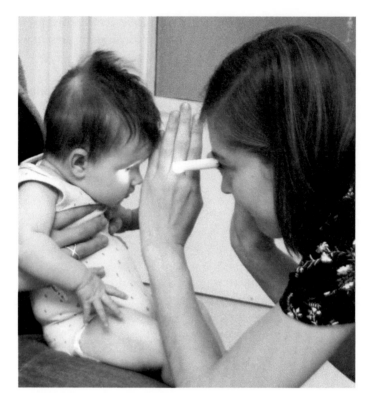

Figure 4.18 Assessment of the pupillary reaction (Item 14) Note that the assessor puts their hand in the midline in order to prevent light being flashed into the contralateral eye.

SCORING

1 = typical	Prompt and symmetric reactions of the eye (pupillary constriction) in which the light is flashed (direct reaction) and of the contralateral eye (indirect, consensual reaction).
0 = atypical	Presence of at least one of the following signs: - no response - slow response, i.e. presence of a delay before response onset and/or a low contraction speed (Hamer et al. 2016) - asymmetric, record atypical side: R/L.

Item 15 Acoustic Reaction to Clapping (T)

POSITION

This item is best assessed in supine (Su) or sitting (Si).

PROCEDURE

Produce a sudden noise by loudly clapping the hands in the vicinity of the infant. Take care not to clap in the infant's visual field and to avoid an airstream toward the infant's face. When the infant does not react to the first stimulus, the procedure should be repeated after at least 10 seconds (e.g. after the assessment of a few other items).

SCORING

1 = typical	Facial reaction, often including blinking of the eyes, turning of the head (Video 4.18). In most typically developing infants the blink reaction habituates after few trials.
0 = atypical	No or doubtful response (Video 4.19).

Note: the presence of an asymmetric facial reaction is scored as a typical response for the acoustic reaction. The asymmetry is recorded as 'atypical' at item 9 (facial appearance).

'MOTOR REACTIONS TO POSTURAL STIMULATION' DOMAIN

Item 16 Pull-to-Sit (T)

POSITION

The starting position of the pull-to-sit manoeuvre is supine (Su).

PROCEDURE

The infant lies in supine position. The examiner takes the infant's wrists in their hand and gently, but not slowly, pulls the infant into a sitting position (Video 4.20). The examiner takes care not to put their thumbs into the hands of the infants, as this facilitates flexor activity in the arms. If the child's head balance is poor, the assessor takes – during traction – both infant's wrists in one hand and uses the other hand to support the infant's head. During traction special attention is paid to the movements of the head, trunk, and arms, and the flexion of the hips. In infants who independently move into a sitting position the pull-to-sit manoeuvre is skipped; the item is assigned score 1.

SCORING

1 = typical	Activates neck and shoulder and arm muscles during traction with symmetric arm activity and adequate hip flexion (Fig. 4.19 and Video 4.20).

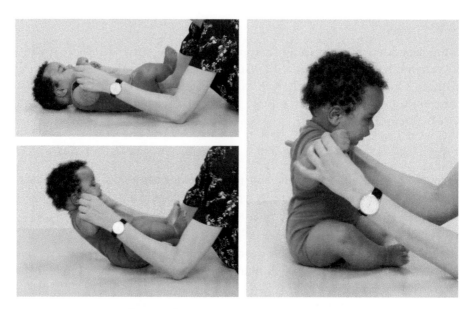

Figure 4.19 Pull–to–sit (Item 16): typical performance in an infant aged 6 months

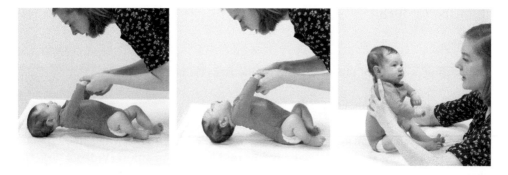

Figure 4.20 Pull–to–sit (Item 16): atypical performance, head lag Head lag during pull–to–sit in an infant aged 2 months.

0 = atypical   Presence of at least one of the following signs:
- head lag (Fig. 4.20 and Video 4.21)
- head in active retroflexion, opisthotonic posture (Fig. 4.21 and Video 4.22)
- no or minimal activation of arm and shoulder muscles, i.e. elbow flexion disappears immediately during traction (Video 4.23)
- inadequate hip flexion (Fig. 4.21 and Video 4.24)
- asymmetric, record atypical side: R/L.

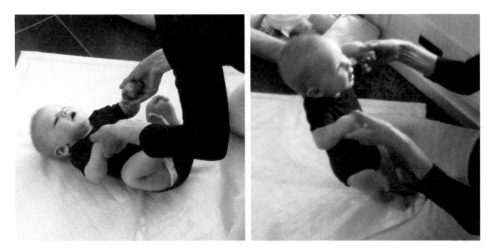

Figure 4.21 **Pull-to-sit (Item 16): atypical performance, inadequate hip flexion**

Item 17 Head in Prone (0)

POSITION

This item is assessed in prone (P).

PROCEDURE

The infant is put in prone position either on an examination table or on a mattress on the floor. The examiner may put the infant's arms in propped position. After placement in prone the infant should not be touched by the examiner. Spontaneous movements of the head are assessed.

SCORING

1 = typical   Lifts head as a selective action allowing for head rotation and/or keeping the head in the midline (Fig. 4.22 and Video 4.25).

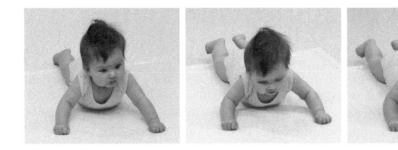

Figure 4.22 **Head in prone (Item 17): typical performance in an infant aged 5 months**

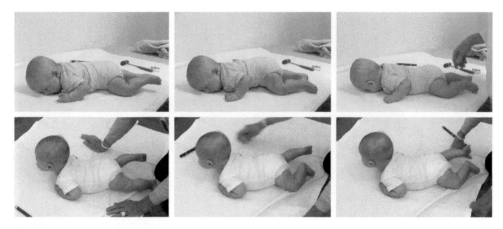

Figure 4.23 Head in prone (Item 17): atypical performance Upper panel: an infant aged 3 months does not lift their head; lower panel: stereotyped hyperextension of neck, limited head rotation in an infant aged 4 months.

0 = atypical Presence of one of the following signs:
      - does not lift head (Fig. 4.23 and Video 4.26)
      - stereotyped hyperextension of the neck, limited head rotation (Fig. 4.23
       and Video 4.27).

Item 18 Prone Suspension   **(T)**

POSITION

This item is assessed in prone suspension (PS).

PROCEDURE

The infant is held in the air in prone position with the examiner's hands around the infant's chest and the limbs hanging free. Movements of neck and trunk are assessed.

SCORING

1 = typical   Keeps the head in line with the trunk or lifts the head higher than the
       trunk level (Fig. 4.24 and Video 4.28).
0 = atypical Presence of at least one of the following signs:
       - head and/or trunk floppy (Fig. 4.25 and Video 4.29)
       - stereotyped, opisthotonus (Fig. 4.26)
       - asymmetric.

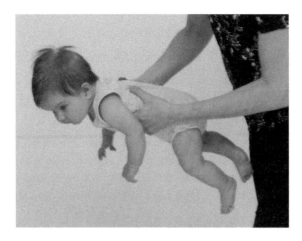

Figure 4.24 Prone suspension (Item 18): typical performance in an infant aged 4 months

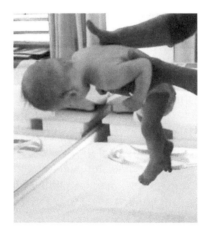

Figure 4.25 Prone suspension (Item 18): atypical performance, floppy head and trunk in an infant aged 8 months

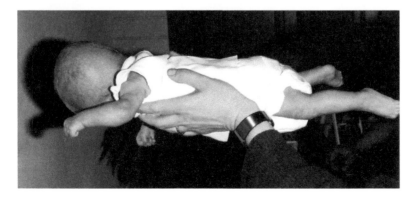

Figure 4.26 Prone suspension (Item 18): atypical performance, stereotyped, opisthotonus

Item 19 Vertical Suspension (T)

Position

This item is assessed in vertical suspension (VS).

Procedure

The examiner holds the infant suspended in vertical position, supporting the infant at the armpits while the examiner's hands hold the infant's upper thorax. Spontaneous movements are assessed for a few seconds, next the infant is gently swung to and fro, both in sideward and forward–backward directions. Movements of head, trunk, and legs are assessed.

Scoring

1 = typical	Head upright and appropriate axillary resistance and varied and symmetric movements of legs (Fig. 4.27 and Video 4.30). Minimal head preference to one side or lateroflexion of the head is considered as typical.
0 = atypical	Presence of at least one of the following signs: - poor head control - slipping through. The slipping through is felt by the assessor. It is also reflected by the observation that the shoulders move to and reach the ears (Fig. 4.28 and Video 4.31) - stereotyped posture or motility of legs, e.g. stereotyped extension with or without 'scissoring', stereotyped floppy leg posture, stereotyped flexion–extension movements, either symmetric or alternating (Fig. 4.29 and Video 4.32) - asymmetric, record atypical side: R/L.

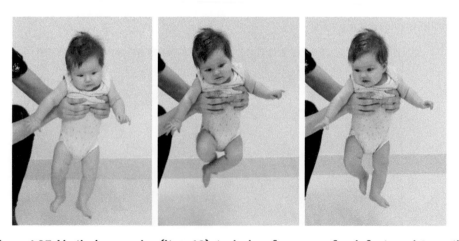

Figure 4.27 Vertical suspension (Item 19): typical performance of an infant aged 4 months

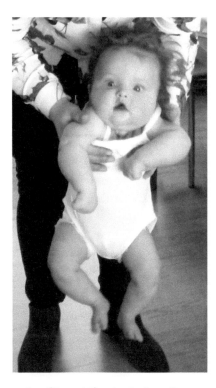

Figure 4.28 Vertical suspension (Item 19): atypical performance, slipping through in an infant aged 5 months

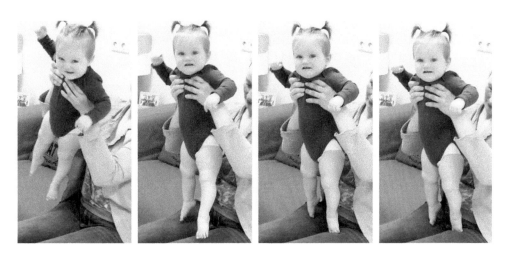

Figure 4.29 Vertical suspension (Item 19): atypical performance, stereotyped behaviour of legs

Item 20 Feet Touching the Ground (T)

POSITION

This item is assessed in vertical suspension (VS).

PROCEDURE

In general, this item is tested immediately after the previous item (Item 19). The starting position is as in Item 19: the examiner holds the infant suspended in vertical position, supporting the infant at the armpits while the examiner's hands hold the infant's upper thorax. Next, the examiner gently lowers the infant so that the feet touch a support surface. The landing on the support surface is repeated two to three times. Movements of the feet are assessed.

SCORING

1 = typical   Varied and symmetric feet postures and movements (Fig. 4.30 and Video 4.33).

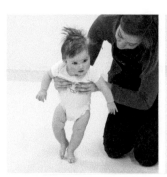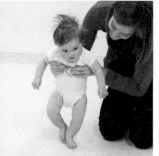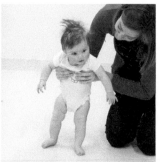

Figure 4.30 Feet touching the ground (Item 20): typical performance

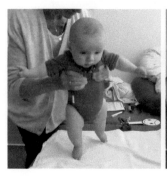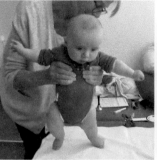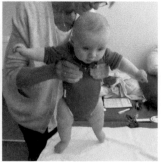

Figure 4.31 Feet touching the ground (Item 20): atypical performance The infant's feet touch the ground with stereotyped tiptoe posturing.

0 = atypical   Presence of stereotyped feet postures, e.g.
- stereotyped plantar flexion (Fig. 4.31 and Video 4.34)
- stereotyped equinovarus
- stereotyped pes valgus
- stereotyped clawing of toes
- asymmetric, record atypical side: R/L.

'MUSCLE TONE' DOMAIN

Not all infants enjoy the assessment of muscle tone. In our experience, the assessment of muscle tone is facilitated when the assessor talks motherese to the infant or sings nursery rhymes.

Item 21 Tone of Neck and Trunk   (T)

POSITION

The muscle tone of neck and trunk is best assessed in supine (Su) or supine suspension (SS) position.

PROCEDURE

The examiner holds the infant in supine position or in supine suspension in front of them, one hand supporting the infant's neck and head, the other supporting the infant's bottom (Fig. 4.32). The infant's head and trunk are gently moved to assess the resistance against passive movements. The passive movements must be carried out with varying velocities and should be repeated several times (Video 4.35). In infants who actively move around this procedure may be skipped; in these infants the item is assigned score 1.

SCORING

1 = typical   Moderate resistance against passive movements.

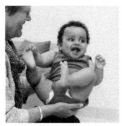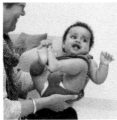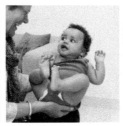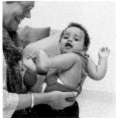

Figure 4.32 Assessment of tone of neck and trunk (Item 21)

0 = atypical   Presence of one of the following signs:
- consistent moderate or severe hypotonia
- consistent moderate or severe hypertonia
- sudden changes in muscle tone, from hypotonia to hypertonia and/ or vice versa.

Item 22 Resistance Against Passive Movements of the Arms, Arm Traction (T)

POSITION

The resistance against passive movements of the arms is best assessed in supine (Su) or sitting (Si) position.

PROCEDURE

In infants who can be assessed easily in supine position, resistance against passive movements of the arms is tested in supine position with the head in midline. Tone in the arms refers to the resistance in passive movements felt across the shoulder, elbow, and wrist joints. The examiner takes the infant's wrist and slowly and gently pulls the infant's arm in vertical position. The examiner takes care not to put their thumbs into the hands of the infant, as this facilitates flexor activity in the arm. The examiner pays special attention to the angle of the elbow. Each arm is tested separately, three times. Thereafter the examiner moves both arms with velocities varying from carefully slow to fast with abrupt changes of movement direction. For the latter manoeuvres both arms may be tested simultaneously (Video 4.36).

In infants who cannot easily be assessed in supine position, which may happen in the second half of the first year, resistance against passive movements of the arms is tested while the infant sits on the parent's lap (Video 4.37). Both arms may be tested simultaneously by moving them with velocities varying from carefully slow to fast with abrupt changes of movement direction.

SCORING

1 = typical   The shoulder remains on the support surface and the elbow shows slight flexion (Fig. 4.33a). Symmetric moderate resistance against passive movements and no change in resistance to fast passive movements.

0 = atypical   Presence of one of the following signs:
- consistent hypotonia, no or very little resistance is felt at shoulder and elbow; the arm is pulled entirely straight (Fig. 4.33b)
- consistent hypertonia, strong resistance is felt at shoulder and elbow, the elbow remains flexed, and it is difficult to move the elbow and

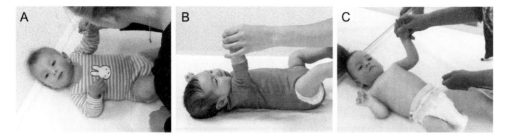

Figure 4.33 Resistance against passive movements of the arms, arm traction (Item 22)
(a) Typical, moderate resistance; (b) hypotonia, the arm is pulled entirely straight; (c) hypertonia, the arm remains flexed/the shoulder is easily lifted from the support surface.

shoulder into another position; the infant's shoulder may be lifted from the support surface (Fig. 4.33c)
- increased resistance at fast passive movements
- sudden changes in muscle tone, from hypotonia to hypertonia and/or vice versa
- asymmetric, record atypical side: R/L.

Item 23 Resistance Against Passive Movements of the Legs, Leg Traction (T)

POSITION

The resistance against passive movements of the legs is best assessed in supine (Su) or sitting (Si) position.

PROCEDURE

In infants who can be assessed easily in supine position, resistance against passive movements of the legs is tested in supine position with the head in midline. Tone in the legs refers to the resistance in passive movements felt across the hip and knee joints. The examiner takes the infant's ankle and slowly and gently pulls the infant's leg in vertical position. The resistance at the angle of the knee and the reaction of the bottom and trunk is assessed. Each leg is tested separately, three times. Thereafter, the examiner moves both legs in hip and knee joint with velocities varying from carefully slow to fast with abrupt changes of movement direction. For the latter manoeuvres both legs may be tested simultaneously (Video 4.38).

In infants who cannot easily be assessed in supine position, which may happen in the second half of the first year, resistance against passive movements of the legs is tested while the infant sits on the parent's lap (Video 4.39). Both legs may be tested

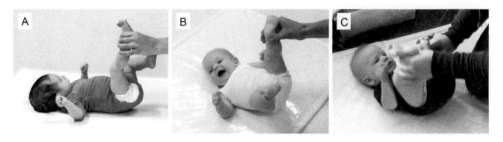

Figure 4.34 Resistance against passive movements of the legs, leg traction (Item 23)
(a) Typical, moderate resistance; (b) hypotonia, the knee is pulled entirely straight; (c) hypertonia, the leg remains markedly flexed/the bottom is easily lifted from the support surface.

simultaneously by moving them with velocities varying from carefully slow to fast with abrupt changes of movement direction.

SCORING

1 = typical	Moderate symmetric resistance against passive movements with moderate knee flexion during pull. The infant's bottom and trunk remain at the support surface (Fig. 4.34a). The resistance does not change in response to fast passive movements.
0 = atypical	Presence of at least one of the following signs:

- consistent hypotonia, no or little resistance is felt at hip and knee is pulled entirely straight (Fig. 4.34b)
- consistent hypertonia, strong resistance is felt at hip and knee, the knee remains markedly flexed, and it is difficult to move the knee into another position; the infant's bottom and trunk may be lifted from the support surface (Fig. 4.34c)
- increased resistance at fast passive movements
- sudden changes in muscle tone, from hypotonia to hypertonia and/ or vice versa
- asymmetric, record atypical side: R/L.

Item 24 Feet: Resistance Against Passive Movements (T)

POSITION

The resistance against passive movements of the feet is best assessed in supine (Su) or sitting (Si) position.

PROCEDURE

The infant lies in supine position or sits on their parent's lap. The infant's head is in midline. One hand of the examiner holds the infant's lower leg, the other hand gently moves the infant's ankle in all directions with abrupt changes of movement direction.

The passive movements must be carried out with various velocities and should be repeated at least three times. Each ankle is tested separately (Video 4.40).

SCORING

1 = typical	Symmetric moderate resistance against passive movements.
0 = atypical	Presence of at least one of the following signs:

- consistent hypotonia, the ankle gives easily way in any direction, with no or little resistance to passive movements
- consistent hypertonia, dorsiflexion to neutral position (90° flexion) difficult or impossible
- increased resistance at fast passive movements
- sudden changes in muscle tone, from hypotonia to hypertonia and/ or vice versa
- asymmetric, record atypical side: R/L (Video 4.41).

'REFLEXES AND REACTIONS' DOMAIN

Item 25 Upper Extremities: Biceps Reflex   (T)

POSITION

The biceps reflex is best assessed in supine (Su) or sitting (Si) position.

PROCEDURE

The infant lies in supine position or sits on their parent's lap. For the evaluation of the biceps reflex the examiner flexes the infant's elbow to 90° to 130°, puts a finger (digit II or III) on the biceps' tendon, while an adjacent finger (the other of digit II and III) is placed on the infant's lower arm. Next, the examiner gently taps the finger resting on the biceps tendon (Fig. 4.35 and Video 4.42). The reaction of the contracting biceps muscle may be felt or seen in the form of a flexion movement of the lower arm. The reflex is evaluated with multiple taps. The taps may be elicited with a reflex hammer or with the examiner's finger. The evaluation focusses on the consistent presence and the consistent symmetry of the response.

SCORING

1 = typical	Symmetric positive response.

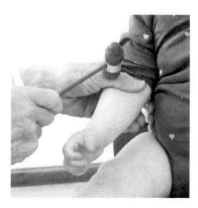

Figure 4.35 Assessment of biceps reflex (Item 25)

0 = atypical   Presence of at least one of the following signs:
- consistently no response, areflexia
- asymmetric, i.e. clear asymmetric response consisting either of the combination of an absent response and a present response, or the combination of a typical response and a clonic response; record atypical side: R/L.

Item 26 Lower Extremities: Knee Jerk and Ankle Clone   (T)

Position

The knee jerk and the ankle clone are best assessed in supine (Su) or sitting (Si) position.

Procedure

The infant lies in supine position or sits on their parent's lap. For the evaluation of the knee jerk the examiner gently lifts the infant's knee in semiflexion. This may be achieved for instance by putting the examiner's middle finger in the popliteal, while their index finger rests on the upper leg just above the knee and their thumb monitors the degree of flexion at the knee. When the examiner feels that the leg is relaxed they tap the patellar tendon (Fig. 4.36 and Video 4.43). The reaction of the contracting quadriceps muscle may be felt or seen in the form of an extension movement of the lower leg. The reflex is evaluated with multiple taps in order to evaluate the consistency of the response. The taps may be elicited with a reflex hammer or with the examiner's finger.

Achilles tendon reflex activity is only evaluated by assessing the presence of ankle clone. To this end the ankle is abruptly moved in dorsiflexion direction (Video 4.43). The presence of ankle clone of at least three beats is noted.

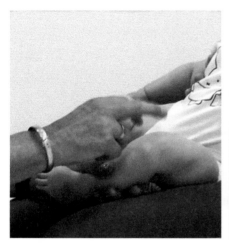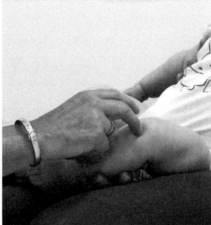

Figure 4.36 Assessment of knee jerk (Item 26)

The evaluation of the tendon reflexes in the lower extremities focusses on the consistent presence of the reaction, the presence of tonic responses in reaction to the knee jerk (Hamer et al. 2018), the presence of clonus, and consistent asymmetries in the responses.

Scoring

1 = typical   Symmetric responses without clonus or tonic reaction.
0 = atypical   Presence of at least one of the following signs:
- consistently no response, areflexia
- tonic reaction; this means the presence of a prolonged contraction of the quadriceps muscle
- clonus
- asymmetric, i.e. clear asymmetric response consisting either of the combination of an absent response and a present response, or the combination of a typical response and a clonic response; record atypical side: R/L.

Item 27 Foot Sole Sensibility   (T)

Position

Foot sole sensibility is best assessed in supine (Su) or sitting (Si) position.

Procedure

The infant lies in supine position or sits on their parent's lap. The examiner gently tickles the foot sole with some of their fingers (Fig. 4.37). Both feet may be assessed

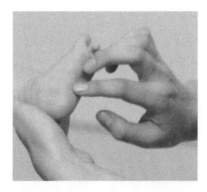

Figure 4.37 Assessment of foot sole sensibility (Item 27) Gentle tickling of the foot sole.

simultaneously or separately. In case of doubt on the presence of asymmetry, the procedure should be repeated.

SCORING

1 = typical	Gentle tickling elicits withdrawal of the leg and varied, symmetrical toe movements (Video 4.44).
0 = atypical	Presence of at least one of the following signs:

- no or virtually no reaction, i.e. the reaction is difficult to observe (Video 4.45)
- stereotyped movements of the toes (Video 4.46)
- asymmetric, i.e. one side clear response, other side no or virtually no response (Video 4.47); record atypical side: R/L.

Item 28 Foot Sole Response   (T)

POSITION

The foot sole response is best assessed in supine (Su) or sitting (Si) position.

PROCEDURE

The infant lies in supine position or sits on their parent's lap. The examiner holds in each hand one of the infant's lower legs between digit II and III. The examiner gently scratches with the nail of their thumb in a continuous movement along the lateral sides of the infant's feet, starting at the metatarsophalangeal joint of the fifth toe and moving to the heel (Fig. 4.38). The responses of the toes are observed. Note the direction of the scratching from toe to heel and not from heel to toe; the latter is the usual way to elicit the response in adults. However, in infants the 'adult' scratching direction may induce an intermingling of foot sole response and plantar grasp reaction.

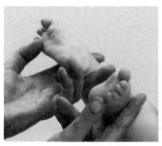 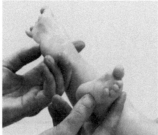 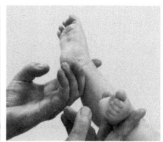

Figure 4.38 Assessment of foot sole response (Item 28) Infant aged 6 months; gently scratching along the lateral side of the infant's foot sole from the toe region to the heel elicits varied movements of the toes.

The scratching procedure is repeated various times. If scratching with moderate intensity does not elicit a response, a slightly higher scratching intensity is applied.

SCORING

1 = typical	Varied dorsiflexion of first toe and toe spreading and symmetric response (Video 4.44).
0 = atypical	Presence of at least one of the following signs:
	- stereotyped, tonic dorsiflexion of first toe (Video 4.48)
	- stereotyped, tonic plantar flexion of first toe, often accompanied by flexion of other toes (Video 4.49)
	- no or virtually no response (Video 4.50)
	- asymmetric, i.e. one side stereotyped response and contralateral side varied or no response, or one side no response and contralateral side varied response (Video 4.51); record atypical side: R/L.

## CHAPTER 5

The Developmental Scale

INTRODUCTION

The Standardized Infant NeuroDevelopmental Assessment (SINDA) developmental scale is a developmental screener for infants aged 6 weeks to 12 months corrected age. It consists of 113 items that are ordered age-wise with 15 items for each month of age, starting at 2 months and ending at 12 months (each month ±2 weeks). Each age-specific set of items consists of items that are relatively easy and items that are relatively difficult for that specific age. The difficult items may return at the following age. This also implies that some items are tested at multiple adjacent ages. The 15 items cover the domains of cognition, communication, and fine and gross motor function. They are scored as pass (1) or fail (0). The number of passed items is added; this results in the infant's developmental score with a maximum of 15.

SINDA's developmental scale consists of two forms, one for the items belonging to the testing ages of 2 to 6 months (Fig. 5.1), the other for the items belonging to the testing ages of 7 to 12 months (Fig. 5.2).

Behavioural State and Testing Situation

Similar to the neurological assessment, an adequate behavioural state is a prerequisite for the developmental assessment (see Chapter 3). This means that the infant should be awake and alert; the infant should not be crying, nor be drowsy or sleeping. At the end of the examination the infant's behavioural state during the assessment is recorded at the top of the form.

Preferably, the infant is assessed in a quiet and child-friendly examination room. The room needs to contain chairs for the parents, an assessment table, a mattress on the floor, and ideally some furniture that may assist pull-to-stand. Specific assessment tools consist of attractive objects to evaluate visual attention and fine motor function, e.g.

Name: .... First name: .... Birth date: .... Ass. date: .... Assessor: .... Hospital: ....

Behavioural state: ☐ awake, alert ☐ sleepy, tired ☐ fussy, moody ☐ crying, cannot be assessed   Corrected age (Mo): ....   ♂ / ♀

Additional clinical comments: ....

1 M 15 - 2 M - 2 M 14

#	Item	Code
1	Smiles in response to smile of parent or assessor	Su / Si
2	Initiates contact with assessor, explores face and facial expression	Su / Si
3	Reacts to cooing-like expressions of parent or assessor	Su / Si
4	Produces ≥2 different sounds (e.g. gaah, ooh)	A
5	Produces sounds as dialogue when being talked to	Su / Si
6	Reacts to sound	A
7	Briefly fixates object at 30cm distance	Su / Si
8	Follows object with eyes or head horizontally	Su / Si
9	Follows object with eyes or head vertically	Su / Si
10	Moves hand to mouth	Su / Si
11	Inspects own hand	Su / Si
12	Moves arm in direction of attractive object	Su / Si
13	Balances head for ≥3 sec in supported sitting	Si
14	Lifts legs alternately on support surface & lifted bilaterally for ≥3 sec	Su
15	Lifts head: chin off support surface for ≥3 sec	P
	Σ	

2 M 15 - 3 M - 3 M 14

#	Item	Code
16	Looks alternately from parents to assessor	Su / Si
4	Produces ≥2 different sounds (e.g. gaah, ooh)	A
5	Produces sounds as dialogue when being talked to	Su / Si
17	Produces sounds with expression: expresses emotions	A
18	Blinks in response to optical approach of hand	Su / Si
19	Turns eyes to sound-producing object	A
20	Turns visual attention slowly from one 'sound object' to another	Su / Si
21	Follows object with eyes or head, horizontally and vertically	Su / Si
11	Inspects own hand	Su / Si
22	Moves arm at appearance of object within visual field	Su / Si
12	Moves arm in direction of attractive object	Su / Si
23	Hands in midline & touching of hands	Su / Si
24	Balances head for ≥5 sec in supported sitting	Si
25	Legs lifted from support surface with ≥3 sec foot-foot contact	Su
26	Lifts head >45° for ≥3 sec	P
	Σ	

3 M 15 - 4 M - 4 M 14

#	Item	Code
16	Looks alternately from parents to assessor	Su / Si
27	Interested in environment and objects in room	A
28	Looks alternately from object to person	Su / Si
29	Produces ≥3 different sounds	A
30	Produces ≥1 labial consonant and one consonant–vowel combination	A
31	Produces sounds to express emotions, laughs loudly	A
20	Turns visual attention slowly from one 'sound object' to another	Su / Si
32	Visually searches to find object that disappeared	Si
12	Moves arm in direction of attractive object	Su / Si
33	Grasps object presented within visual fields with hand	Su / Si
34	Brings object to mouth, & explores with mouth and hand	Su / Si
35	Explores object with both hands	Su / Si
36	Balances head for ≥10 sec in supported sitting, some wobbling allowed	Si
37	Hand touches knee	Su / Si
38	Lifts head >45° with elbow support ≥5 sec	P
	Σ	

4 M 15 - 5 M - 5 M 14

#	Item	Code
27	Interested in environment and objects in room	A
28	Looks alternately from object to person	Su / Si
31	Produces sounds to express emotions, laughs loudly	A
39	Produces ≥3 consonant–vowel combinations	A
40	Localizes voices & directs visual attention to voice	A
32	Visually searches to find object that disappeared	Si
41	Looks ≥3 sec in direction of hidden object	Si
42	Visually explores an object held in their hand	Su / Si
43	Reaches across midline	Su / Si
44	Transfers object from one hand to the other	Su / Si
45	Holds one object & reaches and touches a second one	Su / Si
46	Plays with string	Si
37	Hand touches knee	Su
47	Supported on two elbows & attempts to obtain object	P
48	Stable head position in supported sitting	Si
	Σ	

5 M 15 - 6 M - 6 M 14

#	Item	Code
49	Inspects facial expression of assessor with sustained attention	Su / Si
50	Uses facial expressions to communicate	Su / Si
39	Produces ≥3 consonant–vowel combinations	A
51	Produces sounds to attract attention	A
52	Produces strings of syllables with speech melody	A
53	Turns eyes or head to soft sound, e.g. rustling of paper	A
41	Looks ≥3 sec in direction of hidden object	Si
54	Visually observes falling and 'crashing' object	Si
55	Explores object with interest for details	Su / Si
44	Transfers object from one hand to the other	Su / Si
45	Holds one object & reaches and touches a second one	Su / Si
56	Briefly holds two grasped objects	Su / Si
57	Plays with foot (hand–foot contact)	Su
58	Wriggling	P
59	'Stands' on hands, unilaterally or bilaterally	P
	Σ	

Legend (bottom): ● Interaction ◎ ☺ ⊗ | Emotionality ◎ ☺ ⊗ | Self-Regulation ◎ ☺ ⊗ | React Position ◎ ☺ ⊗ | React Acoustically ◎ ☺ ⊗ | React Visually ◎ ☺ ⊗

Figure 5.1 [displayed on previous page] SINDA developmental and socio-emotional scale assessment form for the ages 6 weeks to 6.5 months The developmental scale has 15 items for each testing month. The testing months range from 2 weeks prior to and 2 weeks later than the actual corrected age in months (as indicated at the top of each item column). The 15 items cover the domains of cognition (indicated on the assessment form with light yellow), communication (dark yellow), fine motor function (green), and gross motor function (blue). The first column at each age contains the item number; the second column the short description of the item; the third column the recommended position of the infant to test the item (A = all positions used during the assessment; P = prone; Si = sitting [independently, with support of the assessor or on the parent's lap]; St = standing; Su = supine); the fourth column is used for scoring: typical performance, i.e. meeting the criteria, is credited with 1 point, atypical performance with a 0. At the bottom the number of credited items is added to form the age-specific developmental score (maximum 15 points). The socio-emotional scale has six items that are presented at the bottom of the form. The item 'interaction' is based on the age-specific items indicated with a red dot. If the infant scores 'typical' on at least half of the interaction items, the interaction item of the socio-emotional scale is classified as typical (happy face icon), otherwise the item is classified as atypical (sad face icon). The items emotionality, self-regulation, and reactivity in response to change of position, reactivity to visual stimuli, and reactivity to acoustic stimuli are scored at the end of the developmental assessment. Scoring is based on the clinical impression of the infant's behaviour during the assessment and consists of a classification as typical (happy face icon) or atypical (sad face icon). Additional clinical details, including the infant's behavioural state, are recorded at the top of the form. A digital version of the form is available online (see access details on page xi).

Name: .... First name: .... Birth date: .... Ass. date: .... Corrected age (mo): .... Hospital: ....

Behavioural state: □ awake, alert □ sleepy, tired □ fussy, moody □ cries, cannot be assessed .... Assessor: .... ♂ / ♀

Additional clinical comments: ....

6 M 15 - **7 M** - 7 M 14	7 M 15 - **8 M** - 8 M 14	8 M 15 - **9 M** - 9 M 14	9 M 15 - **10 M** - 10 M 14	10 M 15 - **11 M** - 11 M 14	11 M 15 - **12 M** - 12 M 14
60 Observes with interest peek-a-boo play — Si ●	60 Observes with interest peek-a-boo play — Si ●	73 Imitates e.g. clapping of hands or waving — Si ●	91 Imitates play of 'clap your hands' or other hand or finger play — Si ●	91 Imitates play of 'clap your hands' or other hand or finger play — Si ●	93 Responds to question: 'Where is..?' (object, person) — A
61 Shows referential gazing — A	73 Imitates e.g. clapping of hands or waving — Si ●	74 Responses to clear 'no' — A ●	92 Uses different expressions or gestures for known and unknown persons — A	82 Responds to own name — A ●	105 Shows semantic gestures when challenged — A
52 Strings of syllables with speech melody — A	52 Strings of syllables with speech melody — A	81 Produces chains of three syllables (canonical babling) — A	82 Responds to own name — A ●	93 Responds to question: 'Where is..?' (object, person) — A ●	106 Uses 'mama' or 'dada' or other meaningful word — A
62 Identifies desires with gestures or facial expressions — A ●	62 Identifies desires with gestures or facial expressions — A ●	82 Responds to own name — A ●	93 Responds to question: 'Where is..?' (object, person) — A ●	94 Produces ≥2 different chains of three syllables — A	95 Looks at pictures in book & turns pages — Si
63 Imitates consonant–vowel sequences — A	63 Imitates consonant–vowel sequences — A	75 Anticipatory gaze to object reappearance — Si	94 Produces ≥2 different chains of three syllables — A	83 Intentionally rings bell — Si	96 Engages in joint exploration (joint attention) — A ●
54 Visually observes falling and 'crashing' object — Si	74 Responses to clear 'no' — Si ●	76 Looks at pictures in book — Si	83 Intentionally rings bell — Si	95 Looks at pictures in book & turns pages — Si	107 Finds object hidden under one of two cups — Si
64 Pays visual attention to scribbling — A	64 Pays visual attention to scribbling — Si	83 Intentionally rings bell — Si	95 Looks at pictures in book & turns pages — Si	96 Engages in joint exploration (joint attention) — A ●	108 Points with index finger to persons or objects — A ●
65 Produces sound by hitting with object — A	75 Anticipatory gaze to object reappearance — A	67 Intentionally pulls string to obtain object — Si	96 Engages in joint exploration (joint attention) — A ●	100 Finds object covered by cup — Si	101 Holds two objects & grasps third object — Si
66 Grasps & holds two objects ≥3 sec — Si	76 Looks at pictures in book — Si	84 Removes obstacle to get object — A	85 Explores details of object with fingertips — A	97 Uses index finger to touch details of object — A	102 Uses spoon to stir in cup or on plate (in imitation) — Si
67 Intentionally pulls string to obtain object — Si	77 Turns object to explore it visually — A	85 Explores details of object with fingertips — Si	86 Puts object in cup — Si	101 Holds two objects & grasps third object — Si	103 Pulls the right string to retrieve object — Si
68 Uses scissor grasp — A	67 Intentionally pulls string to obtain object — Si	86 Puts object in cup — Si	97 Uses index finger to touch details of object — A	102 Uses spoon to stir in cup or on plate (in imitation) — Si	109 Uses pincer grasp — A
69 Sits independently for ≥3 sec — Si	78 Tries to pick object from cup — Si	87 Sits independently for sustained periods of time — Si	88 Sits independently and rotates trunk — Si	103 Pulls the right string to retrieve object — Si	110 Throws small ball forward — Si
70 Turns from supine into prone — Su	69 Sits independently for ≥3 sec — Si	88 Sits independently and rotates trunk — Si	90 Progression on all fours, bunny hop, bottom shuffling — P, Si	90 Progression on all fours, bunny hop, bottom shuffling — P, Si	111 Stands independently for ≥3 sec — Si
71 Reaches out for object in prone — P	79 Gets on all fours independently — Si, P	89 Stands on knees while holding on to furniture — Si	98 Gets into sitting position independently — Su, P	99 Pulls to stand — Si	112 Walks when one hand held — St
72 Pivots — P	80 Progression, e.g. abdominal crawling, rolling — P, Si	90 Progression on all fours, bunny hop, bottom shuffling — P, Si	99 Pulls to stand — A	104 Cruises along furniture — St	113 Squats with support — St
Σ	Σ	Σ	Σ	Σ	Σ

● Interaction ☺ ☹ ⊗ | Emotionality ☺ ☹ ⊗ | Self-Regulation ☺ ☹ ⊗ | React Position ☺ ☹ ⊗ | React Visually ☺ ☹ ⊗ | React Acoustically ☺ ☹ ⊗

Figure 5.2 SINDA developmental and socio-emotional scale assessment form for the ages 6.5 months to 12.5 months For a description see the legends of Figure 5.1. Some items at the oldest ages may also be assessed in Standing (St) position. A digital version of this form is also available online (see access details on page xi).

a Mickey Mouse puppet, a rattle, a picture book, a ball, and two identical-coloured strings (see Fig. 3.1).

Order of the Assessment and Infant Position

The assessment usually starts with the items assessing interaction, as the assessment of these items also promotes the interaction between assessor and infant. The interaction items belong to the cognitive (light yellow) and communication domain (dark yellow), and form the upper part of the age-specific assessment column (see Figs 5.1 and 5.2). Thereafter, the other items of the communication domain follow. The communication domain especially assesses verbal communication (dark yellow). Next, items that assess other cognitive aspects (light yellow), fine motor skills (green), and gross motor skills (blue) follow. The suggested order is not obligatory, though in our experience it is practical and efficient. This also implies that the order in which the items are assessed may be altered when the infant or the situation suggest that another order is better.

We indicated on the form, on the right of the item description, in which positions the items may be assessed most easily. The following abbreviations are used:

- A = all: the item may be tested or observed in any position
- P = prone
- Si = sitting (with or without support)
- St = standing
- Su = supine

In general, the suggested positions are not obligatory, they are meant as practical hints. However, in some items the position is part of the testing item. For instance, Item 13 'Balances head for at least 3 seconds in supported sitting' should be assessed in supported sitting.

General Remarks on the Assessment Form

Each item has a number, starting with the items that emerge at the youngest age. These numbers are used on the form and in the manual. Some items occur only at one testing age; others are present at multiple sequential testing ages. For instance, Item 4 'Produces at least two different sounds (e.g. gaah, ooh)' first appears at 2 months but is repeated at 3 months. In the manual each item is described in normal print at the age at which it first appears; at the ages where the item is repeated the descriptive text is displayed in slightly smaller print, with the remark 'also assessed at age …' as a reminder.

Note that the assessment forms of the developmental scale also serve for the recording of the socio-emotional scale items (at the bottom of the forms). Some developmental items are therefore marked with a red dot: •. The red dot means that the item involves interaction and that the item is also used to assess 'interaction' of the socio-emotional scale (see Chapter 6).

The rest of this chapter describes in detail the standardized assessment and evaluation of all items. As the items are scored as 'pass' or 'fail', the description of items generally only contains the description of the typical 'pass' performance. 'Fail' means that the criteria of typical performance are not met.

The '&' sign on the assessment form denotes that the criteria that are connected by the '&' sign both need to be fulfilled; a comma between options denotes alternatives, not obligatory combinations.

Interpretation of the Results

Addition of the age-specific set of item scores results in SINDA's developmental score. The maximum score is 15 points. A score of ≤7 is considered atypical. If an infant scores atypical we recommend testing the set of items of the adjacent 'younger' column in order to get an impression of the infant's developmental level. Likewise, when an infant achieves 14 or 15 points, the items of the neighbouring 'older' column may be tested to get an idea of the infant's advanced development. Clinically, lower scores are more relevant than higher scores, as an atypical score is associated with intellectual abilities at the age of at least 2 years (Hadders-Algra et al. 2020). Further details on the interpretation of the developmental score are discussed in Chapter 7.

DESCRIPTION OF THE DEVELOPMENTAL ITEMS TESTED AT 2 MONTHS

Item 1•   Smiles in Response to Smile of Parent or Assessor

POSITION

This item is preferably tested in supine (Su) or supported sitting (Si).

PROCEDURE

The assessor smiles multiple times to the infant from a distance of 20cm to 40cm. They do *not* vocalize while smiling. The assessor observes the infant's facial expressions.

RECORDING

Typical performance means that the infant smiles in response (Fig. 5.3 and Video 5.1).

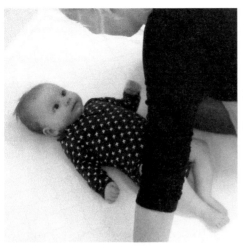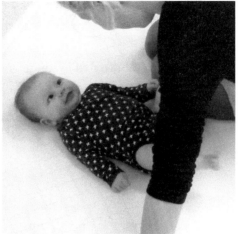

Figure 5.3 Infant smiles in response (Item 1)

Item 2• Initiates Contact With Assessor, Explores Face and Facial Expression

Position

This item is preferably tested in supine (Su) or supported sitting (Si).

Procedure

The assessor or parent looks in the direction of the infant with a friendly expression. The assessor observes the infant's visual behaviour.

Recording

Typical performance means that the infant directs their visual attention to the assessor or parent and visually explore the face and facial expression of the assessor or parent (Fig. 5.4 and Video 5.2).

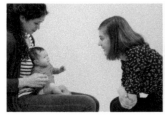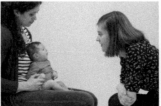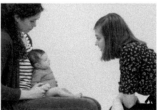

Figure 5.4 Initiates contact with assessor, explores face and facial expression (Item 2•)
Infant aged 2 months communicates with assessor and is interested in their face.

Item 3• Reacts to Cooing-Like Expressions of the Parent or Assessor

Position

This item is preferably tested in supine (Su) or supported sitting (Si).

Procedure

The assessor or parent addresses the infant multiple times with friendly, cooing-like expressions. The assessor observes the infant's motor behaviour, direction of gaze, facial expression, and sounds (Video 5.3).

Recording

Typical performance means that in response to the cooing-like expressions the infant changes their motor behaviour, direction of gaze, or facial expression, with the facial expression reflecting an improvement of mood. The infant may also coo in response.

Item 4 Produces at Least Two Different Sounds, e.g. Gaah or Ooh

Position

This item may be assessed in all positions (A).

Procedure

During the entire assessment the assessor pays attention to the infant's sounds.

Recording

Typical performance means that the infant produces two different sounds, such as gaah, oh, ehh, or u (Video 5.4).

Item 5• Produces Sounds as Dialogue When Being Talked To

Position

This item is preferably tested in supine (Su) or supported sitting (Si).

Procedure

The assessor or the parent talks in a friendly way to the infant, pausing every now and then to allow the infant to respond. The assessor pays attention to the infant's sounds.

Typical performance means that the infant produces sounds in response to being talked to. The response occurs within a few seconds after the words of the assessor or parent (Video 5.4).

Item 6 Reacts to Sound

Position

This item may be assessed in all positions (A).

Procedure

The assessor rings a bell or shakes a rattle twice on each side of the infant's body, out of the infant's view. The assessor observes the infant's behaviour (Fig. 5.5).

Recording

Typical performance means that within a few seconds the infant changes behaviour in response to the sounds, e.g. increases or decreases movement activity, smiles, or cries (Video 5.5).

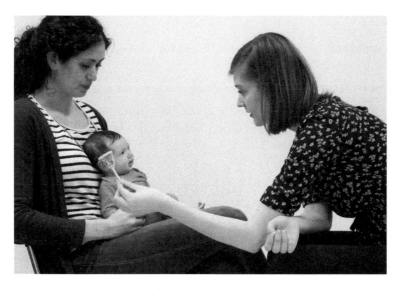

Figure 5.5 Reacts to sound (Item 6) Testing situation in a 2-month-old infant. The assessor engages with the infant and while the infant is paying attention to the assessor, the assessor produces sound with the rattle, which is out of the infant's view.

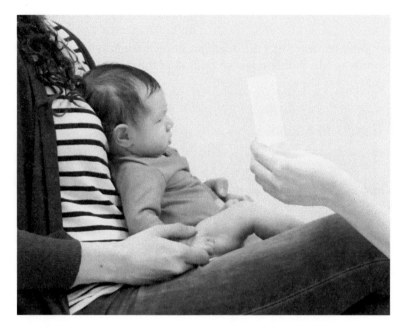

Figure 5.6 Briefly fixates object at 30cm distance (Item 7) Infant aged 2 months fixates the bull's eye.

Item 7   Briefly Fixates Object at 30cm Distance

POSITION

This item is preferably tested in supine (Su) or supported sitting (Si).

PROCEDURE

The assessor holds an attractive object at about 30cm distance within the infant's visual field. Next, the assessor moves the object slowly to and fro. The assessor observes the infant's visual behaviour (Fig. 5.6).

RECORDING

Typical performance means that the infant moves their eyes in the direction of the object and briefly (i.e. for about 1 second) fixates the object (Video 5.6).

Item 8   Follows Object With Eyes or Head Horizontally

POSITION

This item is preferably tested in supine (Su) or supported sitting (Si).

PROCEDURE

The assessor holds an attractive object that does not produce sound at about 30cm distance within the infant's visual field. Next, the assessor slowly and horizontally moves the object, to the right and to the left. Then they repeat this movement sequence. The assessor observes the infant's visual behaviour and head movements.

RECORDING

Typical performance means that the infant horizontally moves the eyes or head in the direction of the object, both to the right and to the left side (Video 5.6).

Item 9   Follows Object With Eyes or Head Vertically

POSITION

This item is preferably tested in supine (Su) or supported sitting (Si).

PROCEDURE

The assessor holds an attractive object that does not produce sound at about 30cm distance within the infant's visual field. Next, the assessor slowly and vertically moves the object, upwards and downwards. Then they repeat this movement sequence. The assessor observes the infant's visual behaviour and head movements.

RECORDING

Typical performance means that the infant vertically moves the eyes or head in the direction of the object, both in the upward and downward direction (Video 5.6).

Item 10   Moves Hand to Mouth

POSITION

This item is preferably tested in supine (Su) or supported sitting (Si).

PROCEDURE

During the assessment the assessor observes the infant's hand movements. If the infant has not brought the hands to the mouth while in supine position or while sitting on the parent's lap, the parent is asked to hold the infant in their arms; the assessor observes whether the infant moves the hand to the mouth in this position.

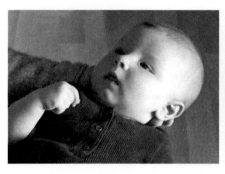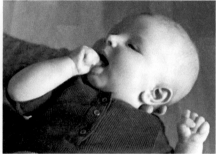

Figure 5.7 Moves hand to mouth (Item 10) Infant aged 2 months.

RECORDING

Typical performance means that the infant moves one or both hands to the mouth so that the hand touches the mouth (Fig. 5.7 and Video 5.7).

Item 11   Inspects Own Hand

POSITION

This item is preferably tested in supine (Su) or supported sitting (Si).

PROCEDURE

During the assessment the assessor observes the infant's hand movements and the infant's visual behaviour. The hand movements are part of the infant's spontaneous movements.

RECORDING

Typical performance means that the infant moves the hands and visually inspects the movements of at least one hand (Fig. 5.8 and Video 5.8).

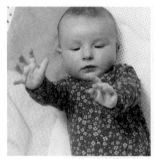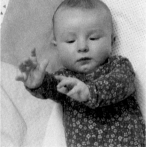

Figure 5.8 Inspects own hand (Item 11)

Atypical performance means that the infants does not move the hands or does not visually inspect one of the moving hands.

Item 12   Moves Arm in Direction of Attractive Object

POSITION

This item is preferably tested in supine (Su) or supported sitting (Si).

PROCEDURE

The assessor presents an attractive object at reaching distance within the infant's visual field. The infant's arms are free to move. The assessor observes the infant's arm and hand movements.

RECORDING

Typical performance means that the infant moves one or both arms in the direction of the object (Fig. 5.9 and Video 5.9).

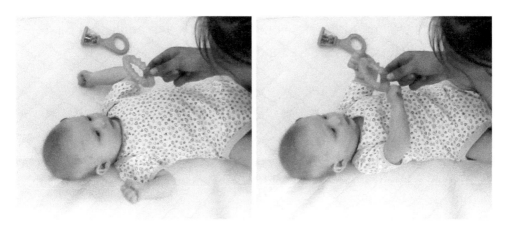

Figure 5.9 Moves arm in direction of attractive object (Item 12)

Item 13   Balances Head for at Least 3 Seconds in Supported Sitting

POSITION

This item is assessed during supported sitting (Si).

PROCEDURE

The assessor puts the infant in sitting position on the assessment mattress while stabilizing the infant's trunk with their hands. The assessor observes the infant's head and trunk movements.

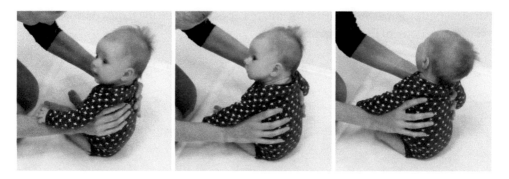

Figure 5.10 Balances head for at least 3 seconds in supported sitting (Item 13)

RECORDING

Typical performance means that the infant is able to balance the head for at least 3 seconds. Wobbling of the head is permitted (Fig. 5.10 and Video 5.10).

Item 14   Lifts Legs Alternately on Support Surface and Lifted Bilaterally for at Least 3 Seconds

POSITION

This item is assessed in supine (Su).

PROCEDURE

During the assessment the assessor observes the infant's leg movements in supine position.

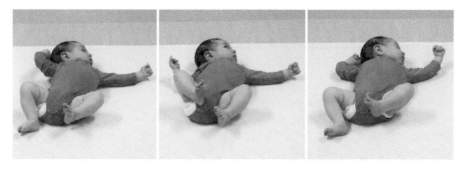

Figure 5.11 Lifts legs alternately on support surface and lifted bilaterally for at least 3 seconds (Item 14)

RECORDING

Typical performance means that the infant alternately lifts the legs from the support surface and puts them down again. In addition, the infant lifts both legs for 3 seconds at least once (Fig. 5.11 and Video 5.11).

Item 15   Lifts Head: Chin off Support Surface for at Least 3 Seconds

POSITION

This item is assessed in prone (P).

PROCEDURE

The assessor puts the infant in prone position with both shoulders in slight adduction and both elbows in flexion with the hands approximately in line with the ears (Fig. 5.12). The assessor observes the infant's head movements.

RECORDING

Typical performance means that the infant lifts the head to such an extent that the chin is off the support surface for at least 3 seconds (Fig. 5.12 and Video 5.12).

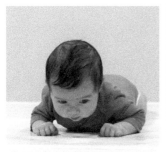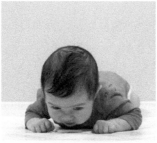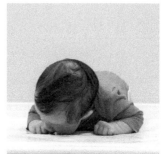

Figure 5.12 Lifts Head: chin off support surface for at least 3 seconds (Item 15) Infant aged 2 months manages to keep the head lifted for at least 3 seconds.

DESCRIPTION OF THE DEVELOPMENTAL ITEMS TESTED AT 3 MONTHS

Item 16●   Looks Alternately From Parents to Assessor

POSITION

This item is preferably tested in supine (Su) or supported sitting (Si).

PROCEDURE

The assessor and parent look with a friendly expression in the direction of the infant; they alternately talk briefly to the infant. Next, they continue their friendly look but keep silent. The assessor observes the infant's visual behaviour.

RECORDING

Typical performance means that – when the parent and assessor stop talking – the infant alternately looks to the parent and assessor (Video 5.13).

Item 4   Produces at Least Two Different Sounds, e.g. Gaah or Ooh –
Also Assessed at 2 Months

POSITION

This item may be assessed in all positions (A).

PROCEDURE

During the entire assessment the assessor pays attention to the infant's sounds.

RECORDING

Typical performance means that the infant produces two different sounds, such as gaah, oh, ehh, or u (Video 5.4).

Item 5•   Produces Sounds as Dialogue When Being Talked to –
Also Assessed at 2 Months

POSITION

This item is preferably tested in supine (Su) or supported sitting (Si).

PROCEDURE

The assessor or the parent talks in a friendly way to the infant. They pause every now and then to allow the infant to respond. The assessor pays attention to the infant's sounds.

RECORDING

Typical performance means that the infant produces sounds in response to being talked to. The response occurs within a few seconds after the words of the assessor (Video 5.4).

Item 17•   Produces Sounds With Expression: Expresses Emotions

POSITION

This item may be assessed in all positions (A).

PROCEDURE

During the assessment the assessor pays attention to the infant's sounds and facial expressions.

RECORDING

Typical performance means that the infant produces sounds with different tonalities and with various facial expressions in accordance with the infant's mood, for instance fear, frustration, and joy (Video 5.14).

Item 18   Blinks in Response to Optical Approach of Hand

POSITION

This item is preferably tested in supine (Su) or supported sitting (Si).

PROCEDURE

The assessor visually engages the infant with their gaze the infant's visual engagement. When the infant is visually engaged, the assessor moves their hand quickly to the infant's eyes. Care is taken not to produce a current of air. The assessor observes the behaviour of the infant's eyes (Fig. 5.13).

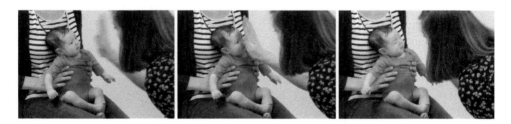

Figure 5.13 Blinks in response to optical approach of hand (Item 18)

RECORDING

Typical performance means that the infant blinks within 1 to 2 seconds (Video 5.15).

Item 19   Turns Eyes to Sound-Producing Object

POSITION

This item may be assessed in all positions (A).

PROCEDURE

The assessor rings a bell or shakes a rattle laterally to the infant's head, out of the infant's view. They repeat this procedure twice on each side of the head. The assessor observes the infant's visual behaviour.

RECORDING

Typical performance means that – within a few seconds – the infant moves their eyes in the direction of the sound-producing object (Video 5.16). To obtain credit for the item the infant only needs to direct the eyes to the sound on one side of the body.

Note: in case of consistent asymmetric reaction consider the presence of an unilateral hearing impairment.

Item 20   Turns Visual Attention Slowly From One 'Sound Object' to Another

POSITION

This item is preferably tested in supine (Su) or supported sitting (Si).

PROCEDURE

The assessor rings a bell or shakes a rattle laterally to the infant's head, out of the infant's view. They repeat this procedure twice on each side of the head (Fig. 5.14). The assessor observes the infant's visual behaviour.

RECORDING

Typical performance means that the infant alternately moves the eyes or the head in the direction of the 'sound objects', and briefly pays visual attention to the source of the sound, at least twice on both sides (Fig. 5.14 and Video 5.17).

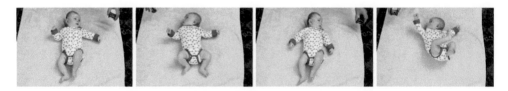

Figure 5.14 Turns visual attention slowly from one 'sound object' to another (Item 20)
A bell or rattle is rung alternately on the left and the right side of the infant's head; this sequence is repeated.

Item 21   Follows Object With Eyes or Head, Horizontally and Vertically

POSITION

This item is preferably tested in supine (Su) or supported sitting (Si).

PROCEDURE

The assessor holds an attractive object that does not produce sound at about 30cm distance within the infant's visual field. Next, they slowly and horizontally move the object, alternately twice to the right and twice to the left, and vertically, twice upwards and twice downwards. The assessor observes the infant's visual behaviour and head movements (Fig. 5.15 and Video 5.18).

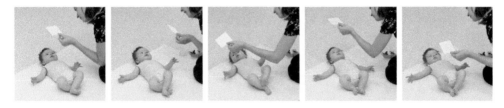

Figure 5.15 Follows object with eyes or head, horizontally and vertically (Item 21)

RECORDING

Typical performance means that the infant horizontally and vertically moves the eyes or head in the direction of the object. This means that the infant moves the eyes or head in all directions, i.e. to the left, the right, and upwards and downwards.

Item 11   Inspects Own Hand – Also Assessed at 2 Months

POSITION

This item is preferably tested in supine (Su) or supported sitting (Si).

PROCEDURE

During the assessment the assessor observes the infant's hand movements and the infant's visual behaviour. The hand movements are part of the infant's spontaneous movements.

RECORDING

Typical performance means that the infant moves the hands and visually inspects the movements of at least one hand (Fig. 5.8 and Video 5.8).

Atypical performance means that the infant does not move the hands, or does not visually inspect one of the moving hands.

Item 22   Moves Arm at Appearance of Object Within Visual Field

POSITION

This item is preferably tested in supine (Su) or supported sitting (Si).

PROCEDURE

The assessor presents an attractive, sound-producing object, such as a rattle, at reaching distance within the infant's visual field. The infant's arms are free to move. The assessor observes the infant's arm and hand movements.

RECORDING

Typical performance means that the infant increases motility of one or both arms and one or both hands in response to object presentation (Video 5.19).

Item 12   Moves Arm in Direction of Attractive Object – Also Assessed at 2 Months

POSITION

This item is preferably tested in supine (Su) or supported sitting (Si).

PROCEDURE

The assessor presents an attractive object at reaching distance within the infant's visual field. The infant's arms are free to move. The assessor observes the infant's arm and hand movements.

RECORDING

Typical performance means that the infant moves one or both arms in the direction of the object (Fig. 5.9 and Video 5.9).

Item 23   Hands in Midline and Touching of Hands

POSITION

This item is preferably tested in supine (Su) or supported sitting (Si).

PROCEDURE

During the assessment the assessor observes the infant arm and hand movements.

RECORDING

Typical performance means that the infant moves both hands to the midline, where the hands touch (Fig. 5.16 and Video 5.20).

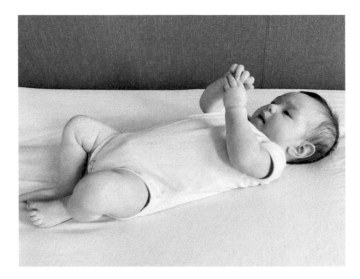

Figure 5.16 Hands in midline and touching of hands (Item 23)

Item 24 Balances Head for at Least 5 Seconds in Supported Sitting

Position

This item is assessed during supported sitting (Si).

Procedure

The assessor puts the infant in sitting position on the assessment mattress while stabilizing the infant's trunk with their hands. The assessor observes the infant's head and trunk movements.

Recording

Typical performance means that the infant keeps the head upright for at least 5 seconds. Wobbling head movements are allowed (Video 5.21).

Item 25 Legs Lifted From Support Surface With at Least 3 Seconds Foot–Foot Contact

Position

This item is assessed in supine (Su).

Procedure

During the assessment the assessor observes the infant's leg movements in supine position.

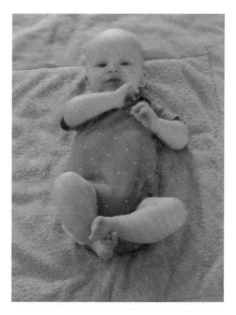

Figure 5.17 Legs lifted from support surface with at least 3 seconds foot–foot contact (Item 25)

RECORDING

Typical performance means that the infant lifts the legs from the support surface and in this position the feet touch for at least 3 seconds (Fig. 5.17 and Video 5.22).

Item 26   Lifts Head Over 45° for at Least 3 Seconds

POSITION

This item is assessed in prone (P).

PROCEDURE

The assessor puts the infant in prone position with both shoulders in slight adduction and both elbows in flexion with the hands approximately in line with the ears. The assessor observes the infant's head and trunk movements.

RECORDING

Typical performance means that the infant lifts the head over 45° for at least 3 seconds (Fig. 5.18 and Video 5.23).

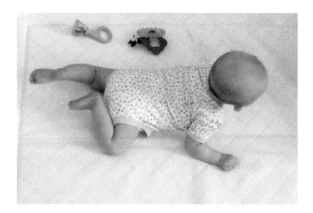

Figure 5.18 Lifts head over 45° for at least 3 seconds (Item 26)

DESCRIPTION OF THE DEVELOPMENTAL ITEMS TESTED AT 4 MONTHS

Item 16• Looks Alternately From Parents To Assessor – Also Assessed at 3 Months

POSITION

This item is preferably tested in supine (Su) or supported sitting (Si).

PROCEDURE

The assessor and parent look with a friendly expression in the direction of the infant; they alternately talk briefly to the infant. Next, they continue to look with a friendly expression but keep silent. The assessor observes the infant's visual behaviour.

RECORDING

Typical performance means that – when the parent and assessor stopped talking – the infant alternately looks to the parent and assessor (Video 5.13).

Item 27• Interested in Environment and Objects in Room

POSITION

This item may be assessed in all positions (A).

PROCEDURE

During the assessment the assessor observes the infant's visual behaviour.

RECORDING

Typical performance means that the infant looks around with interest for a prolonged period (Video 5.24).

Item 28•   Looks Alternately From Object to Person

POSITION

This item is preferably tested in supine (Su) or supported sitting (Si).

PROCEDURE

The assessor or the parent presents an attractive object to the infant. Next, the assessor or the parent talks to the infant. The assessor observes the infant's visual attention.

RECORDING

Typical performance means that the infant turns visual attention from the object to the person (Video 5.25).

Item 29   Produces at Least Three Different Sounds

POSITION

This item may be assessed in all positions (A).

PROCEDURE

During the assessment the assessor pays attention to the infant's sounds.

RECORDING

Typical performance means that the infant produces at least three different sounds (Video 5.26).

Item 30   Produces at Least One Labial Consonant and One Consonant–Vowel Combination

POSITION

This item may be assessed in all positions (A).

PROCEDURE

During the assessment the assessor pays attention to the infant's sounds.

RECORDING

Typical performance means that the infant produces one labial consonant (m, b, p, f, v) and at least one consonant–vowel combination (e.g. ba, ma). All potential vowels may be uttered (Video 5.27).

Item 31• Produces Sounds to Express Emotions, Laughs Loudly

POSITION

This item may be assessed in all positions (A).

PROCEDURE

During the assessment the assessor pays attention to the infant's sounds and facial expressions.

RECORDING

Typical performance means that the infant produces sounds in different tonalities with various facial expressions in accordance with the infant's mood, for instance fear, frustration, and joy. The repertoire of sounds may also include clearly audible laughing (Video 5.28).

Item 20 Turns Visual Attention Slowly From One 'Sound Object' to Another – Also Assessed at 3 Months

POSITION

This item is preferably tested in supine (Su) or supported sitting (Si).

PROCEDURE

The assessor holds a sound-producing object such as a bell or rattle on both sides of the infant's head, out of the infant's view (Fig. 5.14). They alternately ring/shake them. This procedure is repeated twice. The assessor observes the infant's visual behaviour.

RECORDING

Typical performance means that the infant alternately moves the eyes or the head in the direction of the 'sound objects', and briefly pays visual attention to the source of the sound, at least twice on both sides (Video 5.17).

Item 32 Visually Searches to Find Object That Disappeared

POSITION

This item is assessed during supported sitting (Si).

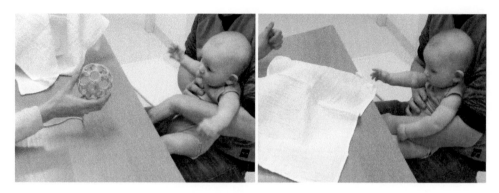

Figure 5.19 Visually searches to find object that disappeared (Item 32)

PROCEDURE

The assessor attracts the infant's attention to an attractive object on the table. Next, they put a neutral (i.e. non-interesting) cloth near the object. When the infant has lost interest in the cloth, the assessor covers the attractive object with the cloth and observes the infant's visual attention (Fig. 5.19).

RECORDING

Typical performance means that the infant briefly gives visual attention to the covered object (Video 5.29).

Item 12   Moves Arm in Direction of Attractive Object – Also Assessed at 2 and 3 Months

POSITION

This item is preferably tested in supine (Su) or supported sitting (Si).

PROCEDURE

The assessor presents an attractive object at reaching distance within the infant's visual field. The infant's arms are free to move. The assessor observes the infant's arm and hand movements.

RECORDING

Typical performance means that the infant moves one or both arms in the direction of the object (Fig. 5.9 and Video 5.9).

Item 33   Grasps Object Presented Within Visual Field With Hand

POSITION

This item is preferably tested in supine (Su) or supported sitting (Si).

PROCEDURE

The assessor presents an attractive object, such as a rattle or a Mickey Mouse toy, within the visual field at reaching distance in the midline. When the infant does not grasp the toy, the object is presented more laterally, in the infant's right and left visual field. The assessor observes the infant's arm and hand movements.

RECORDING

Typical performance means that the infant grasps the object with one or two hands (Fig. 5.20 and Video 5.30).

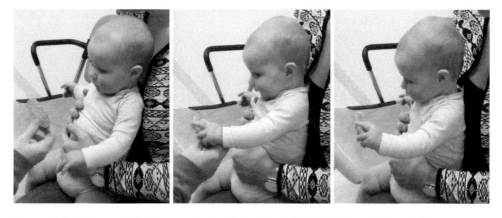

Figure 5.20 Grasps object presented within visual field with hand (Item 33)

Item 34   Brings Object to Mouth, and Explores With Mouth and Hand

POSITION

This item is preferably tested in supine (Su) or supported sitting (Si).

PROCEDURE

The assessor presents an attractive object at reaching distance in the midline. When the infant does not grasp the toy, the object is presented more laterally in

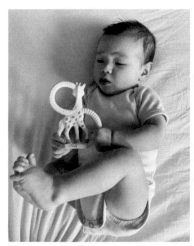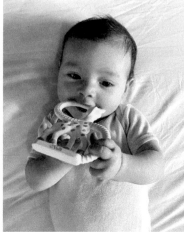

Figure 5.21 Brings object to mouth, and explores with mouth and hand (Item 34)

the infant's right and left visual field. The assessor observes the infant's arm and hand movements.

RECORDING

Typical performance means that the infant grasps the object with one or two hands and brings it to the mouth and explores the object with the mouth and one or two hands (Fig. 5.21 and Video 5.31).

Item 35   Explores Object With Both Hands

POSITION

This item is preferably tested in supine (Su) or supported sitting (Si).

PROCEDURE

The assessor presents an attractive object at reaching distance within the infant's visual field. The assessor observes the infant's arm and hand movements.

RECORDING

Typical performance means that the infant grasps the object and explores it with both hands (with the hands only, not simultaneously with the mouth) (Fig. 5.22 and Video 5.32).

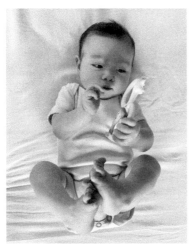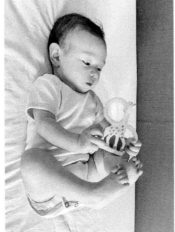

Figure 5.22 Explores object with both hands (Item 35)

Item 36 Balances Head for at Least 10 Seconds in Supported Sitting, Some Wobbling Allowed

POSITION

This item is assessed during supported sitting (Si).

PROCEDURE

The assessor puts the infant in sitting position on the assessment mattress while stabilizing the infant's trunk with their hands. The assessor observes the infant's head and trunk movements.

RECORDING

Typical performance means that the infant keeps the head upright for at least 10 seconds. Some wobbling is allowed (Video 5.33).

Item 37 Hand Touches Knee

POSITION

This item is assessed in supine (Su).

PROCEDURE

During the assessment the assessor observes the infant's arm and leg movements.

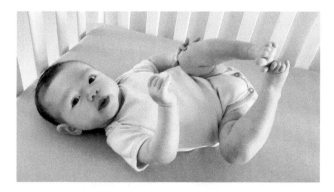

Figure 5.23 Hand touches knee (Item 37)

RECORDING

Typical performance means that the infant lifts both legs from the support surface and touches one knee with at least one hand (Fig. 5.23 and Video 5.34).

Item 38   Lifts Head Over 45° With Elbow Support for at Least 5 Seconds

POSITION

This item is assessed in prone (P).

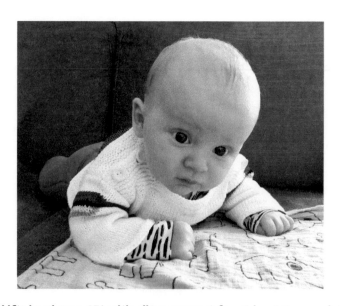

Figure 5.24 Lifts head over 45° with elbow support for at least 5 seconds (Item 38)

PROCEDURE

The assessor puts the infant in prone position with both shoulders in slight adduction and both elbows in flexion with the hands approximately in line with the ears. The assessor observes the infant's head, trunk, and arm movements.

RECORDING

Typical performance means that the infant lifts the head over 45° and for at least 5 seconds uses the support of the lower arms (so-called 'elbow support') to stabilize position (Fig. 5.24 and Video 5.35).

DESCRIPTION OF THE DEVELOPMENTAL ITEMS TESTED AT 5 MONTHS

Item 27• Interested in Environment and Objects in Room – Also Assessed at 4 Months

POSITION

This item may be assessed in all positions (A).

PROCEDURE

During the assessment the assessor observes the infant's visual behaviour.

RECORDING

Typical performance means that the infant looks around with interest for a prolonged period (Video 5.24).

Item 28• Looks Alternately From Object to Person – Also Assessed at 4 Months

POSITION

This item is preferably tested in supine (Su) or supported sitting (Si).

PROCEDURE

The assessor or the parent presents an attractive object to the infant. Next, the assessor or the parent talks to the infant. The assessor observes the infant's visual attention.

RECORDING

Typical performance means that the infant turns visual attention from the object to the person (Video 5.25).

Item 31• Produces Sounds to Express Emotions, Laughs Loudly – Also Assessed at 4 Months

POSITION

This item may be assessed in all positions (A).

PROCEDURE

During the assessment the assessor pays attention to the infant's sounds and facial expressions.

RECORDING

Typical performance means that the infant produces sounds in different tonalities with various facial expressions in accordance with the infant's mood, for instance fear, frustration, and joy. The repertoire of sounds may also include clearly audible laughing (Video 5.28).

Item 39 Produces at Least Three Consonant–Vowel Combinations

POSITION

This item may be assessed in all positions (A).

PROCEDURE

During the assessment the assessor pays attention to the vocalizations of the infant.

RECORDING

Typical performance means that the infant produces at least three consonant–vowel combinations. All potential vowels may be uttered (Video 5.36).

Item 40• Localizes Voices and Directs Visual Attention to Voice

POSITION

This item may be assessed in all positions (A).

PROCEDURE

The assessor or the parent is sitting or standing on the infant's side but not within the infant's view. They start to talk to the infant. The assessor observes the infant's visual attention.

Recording

Typical performance means that the infant moves the eyes in the direction of the voice (Video 5.37).

Item 32   Visually Searches to Find Object That Disappeared – Also Assessed at 4 Months

Position

This item is assessed during supported sitting (Si).

Procedure

The assessor attracts the infant's attention to an attractive object on the table. Next, they put a neutral (i.e. non-interesting) cloth near the object. When the infant has lost interest in the cloth, the assessor covers the object with the cloth and observes the infant's visual attention (Fig. 5.19).

Recording

Typical performance means that the infant briefly gives visual attention to the covered object (Video 5.29).

Item 41   Looks for at Least 3 Seconds in the Direction of a Hidden Object

Position

This item is assessed during supported sitting (Si).

Procedure

The assessor puts an attractive object on the table and draws the infant's attention to the object. Next, they cover the object with a neutral (i.e. a non-interesting) cloth and assess the infant's visual attention.

Recording

Typical performance means that the infant looks at least for 3 seconds in the direction of the hidden object (Fig. 5.25 and Video 5.38).

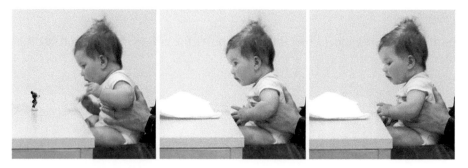

Figure 5.25 **Looks for at least 3 seconds in the direction of a hidden object (Item 41)**

Item 42   Visually Explores an Object Held in Their Hand

POSITION

This item is preferably tested in supine (Su) or supported sitting (Si).

PROCEDURE

The assessor presents an attractive object at reaching distance within the infant's visual field. The assessor observes the infant's visual attention and hand movements.

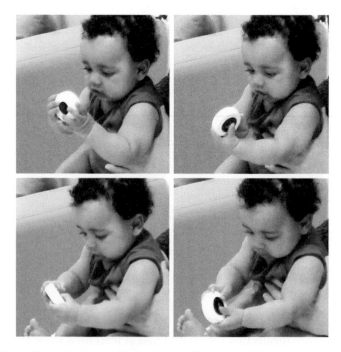

Figure 5.26 **Visually explores an object held in their hand (Item 42)**

Typical performance means that the infant grasps the object. The infant holds the object in at least one hand and explores it visually (Fig. 5.26 and Video 5.39).

Item 43   Reaches Across Midline

POSITION

This item is preferably tested in supine (Su) or supported sitting (Si).

PROCEDURE

The assessor presents an attractive object at reaching distance within the visual field at some distance from the infant's midline, i.e. near the nipple line contralaterally to the reaching arm. The 'non-reaching' ipsilateral arm of the infant may be held by the assessor. The assessor observes the infant's arm and hand movements.

RECORDING

Typical performance means that the infant reaches and may grasp the object by moving the arm – the contralateral one from the point of view of object presentation – across the midline. To pass the criterion, only one arm needs to cross the midline (Fig. 5.27 and Video 5.40).

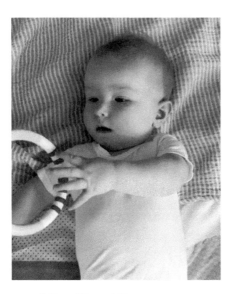

Figure 5.27 Reaches across midline (Item 43)

Item 44   Transfers Object From One Hand to the Other

POSITION

This item is preferably tested in supine (Su) or supported sitting (Si).

PROCEDURE

The assessor presents an attractive object at reaching distance within the infant's visual field. The assessor observes the infant's arm and hand movements.

RECORDING

Typical performance means that the infant grasps the object and transfers it from one hand to the other hand (Fig. 5.28 and Video 5.41).

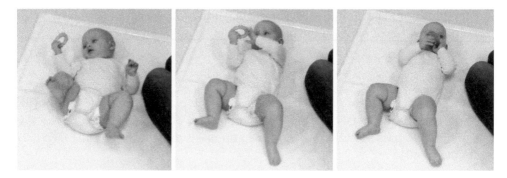

Figure 5.28 Transfers object from one hand to the other (Item 44)

Item 45   Holds One Object and Reaches and Touches a Second One

POSITION

This item is preferably tested in supine (Su) or supported sitting (Si).

PROCEDURE

The assessor presents an attractive object at reaching distance within the infant's visual field. When the infant has grasped the object, the assessor presents a second attractive object. The assessor observes the infant's arm and hand movements.

RECORDING

Typical performance means that the infant grasps and holds the first object. While holding the first object in their hand, they reach with the other hand towards the second

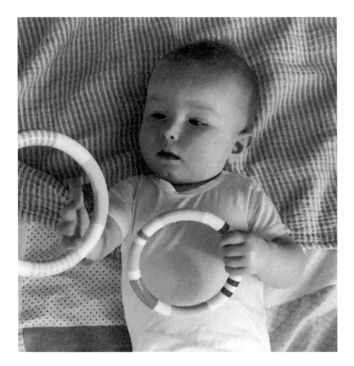

Figure 5.29 Holds one object and reaches and touches a second one (Item 45)

object and touch it. This reaching attempt does not need to result in successful grasping (Fig. 5.29 and Video 5.42).

Item 46   Plays With String

POSITION

This item is assessed during supported sitting (Si).

PROCEDURE

The assessor puts a coloured string on the table at reaching distance within the infant's view. The assessor observes the infant's hand and finger movements.

RECORDING

Typical performance means that the infant moves the string with their fingers (Fig. 5.30 and Video 5.43).

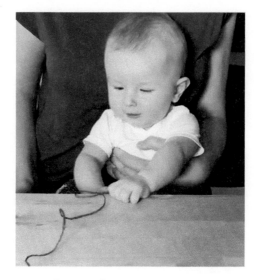

Figure 5.30 Plays with string (Item 46)

Item 37   Hand Touches Knee – Also Assessed at 4 Months

POSITION

This item is assessed in supine (Su).

PROCEDURE

During the assessment the assessor observes the infant's arm and leg movements.

RECORDING

Typical performance means that the infant lifts both legs from the support surface and touches one knee with at least one hand (Fig. 5.23 and Video 5.34).

Item 47   Supported on Two Elbows and Attempts to Obtain Object

POSITION

This item is assessed in prone (P).

PROCEDURE

The assessor puts the infant in prone position with both shoulders in adduction and both elbows in flexion with the hands approximately in line with the ears. They put

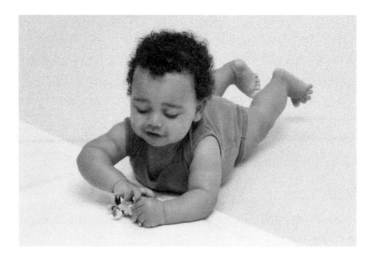

Figure 5.31 Supported on two elbows and attempts to obtain object (Item 47)

an attractive object at reaching distance within the infant's visual field. The assessor observes the infant's arm and hand movements.

Recording

Typical performance means that the infant, who supports themself on both lower arms (so-called 'elbow support'), reaches out for the object. To pass the criterion, reaching does not need to result in grasping (Fig. 5.31 and Video 5.44).

Item 48   Stable Head Position in Supported Sitting

Position

This item is assessed during supported sitting (Si).

Procedure

The assessor puts the infant in sitting position on the assessment mattress while stabilizing the infant's trunk with their hands. The assessor observes the infant's movements of head and trunk.

Recording

Typical performance means that the infant keeps the head upright for at least 10 seconds without wobbling (Video 5.45).

DESCRIPTION OF THE DEVELOPMENTAL ITEMS TESTED AT 6 MONTHS

Item 49• Inspects Facial Expression of Assessor With Sustained Attention

POSITION

This item is preferably tested in supine (Su) or supported sitting (Si).

PROCEDURE

The assessor looks with a friendly expression to the infant. The assessor observes the infant's visual attention.

RECORDING

Typical performance means that the infant visually explores the assessor's facial expression with sustained attention (Video 5.46).

Item 50• Uses Facial Expressions to Communicate

POSITION

This item is preferably tested in supine (Su) or supported sitting (Si).

PROCEDURE

During the assessment the assessor observes the visual behaviour, facial expressions, and gestures of the infant.

RECORDING

Typical performance means that the infant uses visual behaviour, facial expressions, and gestures to initiate communication with parent or assessor (Video 5.47).

Item 39 Produces at Least Three Consonant–Vowel Combinations – Also Assessed at 5 Months

POSITION

This item may be assessed in all positions (A).

PROCEDURE

During the assessment the assessor pays attention to the vocalizations of the infant.

RECORDING

Typical performance means that the infant produces at least three consonant–vowel combinations. All potential vowels may be uttered (Video 5.36).

Item 51• Produces Sounds to Attract Attention

POSITION

This item may be assessed in all positions (A).

PROCEDURE

During the assessment the assessor pays attention to the infant's sounds and to the infant's head, face, and eye movements.

RECORDING

Typical performance means that the infant uses sounds (not crying) to attract the attention of the parent or assessor to themselves (Video 5.48).

Item 52 Produces Strings of Syllables With Speech Melody

POSITION

This item may be assessed in all positions (A).

PROCEDURE

During the assessment, the assessor pays attention to the infant's vocalizations.

RECORDING

Typical performance means that the infant produces strings of syllables with speech melody (variation in pitch and volume), e.g. aionaba, wadabe, gedebe (Video 5.49).

Item 53 Turns Eyes or Head to Soft Sound, e.g. Rustling of Paper

POSITION

This item may be assessed in all positions (A).

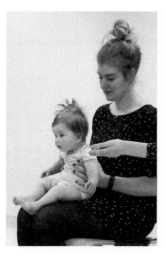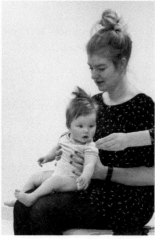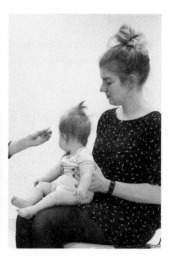

Figure 5.32 Turns eyes or head to soft sound, e.g. rustling of paper (Item 53)

PROCEDURE

The assessor produces a soft sound, e.g. rustling of paper, laterally to the infant, out of their view. First one side is tested, then the other. The assessor observes the infant's head and eye movements.

RECORDING

Typical performance means that the infant moves the eyes or head in the direction of the sound. To pass the criterion it is sufficient that the infant moves the head in one direction only (Fig. 5.32 and Video 5.50).

Item 41   Looks for at Least 3 Seconds in the Direction of a Hidden Object –
Also Assessed at 5 Months

POSITION

This item is assessed during supported sitting (Si).

PROCEDURE

The assessor puts an attractive object on the table and draws the infant's attention to the object. Next, they cover the object with a neutral (i.e. a non-interesting) cloth and assess the infant's visual attention.

RECORDING

Typical performance means that the infant looks at least for 3 seconds in the direction of the hidden object (Fig. 5.25 and Video 5.38).

Item 54   Visually Observes Falling and 'Crashing' Object

POSITION

This item is assessed during supported sitting (Si).

PROCEDURE

The assessor holds an attractive object in the infant's view and waits until the infant has visually explored the object. Next, the assessor drops the object, so that it clatters, i.e. 'crashes'. The assessor observes the infant's visual attention. If the infant does not respond to the first 'crash', the sequence is repeated once more.

RECORDING

Typical performance means that the infant visually follows the 'crashing' object to the floor (Fig. 5.33 and Video 5.51).

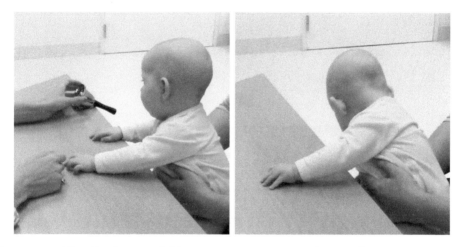

Figure 5.33 Visually observes falling and 'crashing' object (Item 54)

Item 55   Explores Object With Interest for Details

POSITION

This item is preferably tested in supine (Su) or supported sitting (Si).

PROCEDURE

The assessor presents an attractive object with details, such as a car, animal, tiny doll, figure, at reaching distance within the infant's visual field. The assessor observes the infant's hand and finger movements.

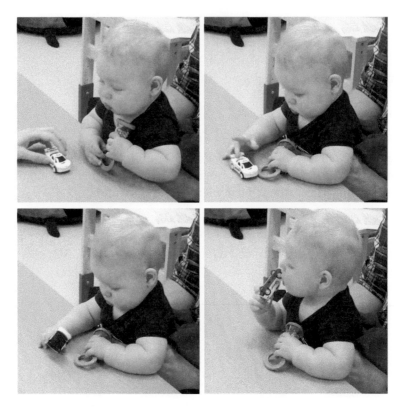

Figure 5.34 Explores object with interest for details (Item 55)

RECORDING

Typical performance means that the infant looks with interest at the object, and explores the details of the object by touching it with the fingers (Fig. 5.34 and Video 5.52).

Item 44   Transfers Object From One Hand to the Other – Also Assessed at 5 Months

POSITION

This item is preferably tested in supine (Su) or supported sitting (Si).

PROCEDURE

The assessor presents an attractive object at reaching distance within the infant's visual field. The assessor observes the infant's arm and hand movements.

Recording

Typical performance means that the infant grasps the object and transfers it from one hand to the other (Fig. 5.28 and Video 5.41).

Item 45 Holds One Object and Reaches and Touches a Second One – Also Assessed at 5 Months

Position

This item is preferably tested in supine (Su) or supported sitting (Si).

Procedure

The assessor presents an attractive object at reaching distance within the infant's visual field. When the infant has grasped the object, the assessor presents a second attractive object. The assessor observes the infant's arm and hand movements.

Recording

Typical performance means that the infant grasps and holds the first object. While holding the first object in their hand, they reach with the other hand towards the second object and touch it. This reaching attempt does not need to result in successful grasping (Fig. 5.29 and Video 5.42).

Item 56 Briefly Holds Two Grasped Objects

Position

This item is preferably tested in supine (Su) or supported sitting (Si).

Procedure

The assessor presents an attractive object at reaching distance within the infant's visual field. When the infant has grasped the object, the assessor presents a second attractive object. The assessor observes the infant's arm and hand movements.

Recording

Typical performance means that the infant grasps and holds the first object. While holding the first object in their hand, they reach with the other hand towards the second object and grasp it. To pass the criterion, the infant only needs to hold both objects momentarily (Fig. 5.35 and Video 5.53).

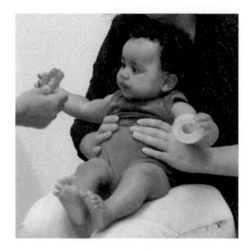

Figure 5.35 **Briefly holds two grasped objects (Item 56)**

Item 57   Plays With Foot (Hand–Foot Contact)

POSITION

This item is assessed in supine (Su).

PROCEDURE

During the assessment the assessor observes the infant's hand and feet movements while in supine.

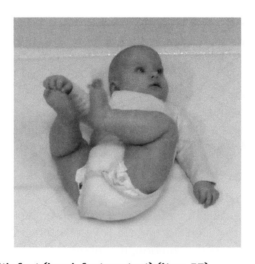

Figure 5.36 **Plays with foot (hand–foot contact) (Item 57)**

RECORDING

Typical performance means that the infant lifts both legs from the support surface and touches one foot with at least one hand (Fig. 5.36 and Video 5.54).

Item 58   Wriggling

POSITION

This item is assessed in prone (P).

PROCEDURE

The assessor puts the infant in prone position with both shoulders in adduction and both elbows in flexion with the hands approximately in line with the ears. The assessor puts an attractive object just out of reaching distance within the infant's visual field. The assessor observes the infant's trunk and extremity movements.

RECORDING

Typical performance means that the infant wriggles. Wriggling movements consist of small, quick, twisting and turning body movements resulting in minor spatial displacements while the abdomen remains in contact with the support surface. Wriggling may result in small backward movements – forward displacement is just minimal (Video 5.55).

Item 59   'Stands' on Hands, Unilaterally or Bilaterally

POSITION

This item is assessed in prone (P).

PROCEDURE

The assessor puts the infant in prone position with both shoulders in slight adduction and both elbows in flexion with the hands approximately in line with the ears. The assessor observes the infant's arm and hand movements.

RECORDING

Typical performance means that the infant supports itself by 'standing' on the hands. The standing implies that the elbow is extended. To pass the criterion, the standing behaviour only needs to be present on one side; the other arm may be involved in other activities such as pointing or grasping (Fig. 5.37 and Video 5.56).

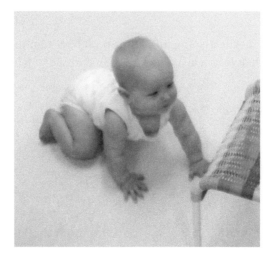

Figure 5.37 'Stands' on hands, unilaterally or bilaterally (Item 59)

DESCRIPTION OF THE DEVELOPMENTAL ITEMS TESTED AT 7 MONTHS

Item 60• Observes With Interest Peek-a-Boo Play

POSITION

This item is assessed during sitting (Si).

PROCEDURE

In order to play peek-a-boo, the assessor engages in visual contact with the infant. Next, the assessor 'hides' their face behind a sheet of paper or behind their hands, before uncovering themselves after a few seconds, saying 'peek-a-boo!'. If the infant does not respond, the procedure is repeated once more. The assessor observes the infant's behaviour.

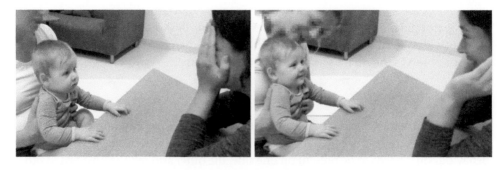

Figure 5.38 Observes with interest peek–a–boo play (Item 60•)

Typical performance means that the infant shows interest in the peek-a-boo play by stopping other activities, directing visual attention to the assessor, changing facial expression, or vocalizing (Fig. 5.38 and Video 5.57).

Item 61• Shows Referential Gazing

POSITION

This item may be assessed in all positions (A).

PROCEDURE

During the assessment the assessor observes the visual attention of the infant, who plays with an object.

RECORDING

Typical performance means that the infant looks at the object, but interrupts this looking behaviour sometimes to look to parent or assessor, after which the infant returns their visual attention to the object (Fig. 5.39 and Video 5.58).

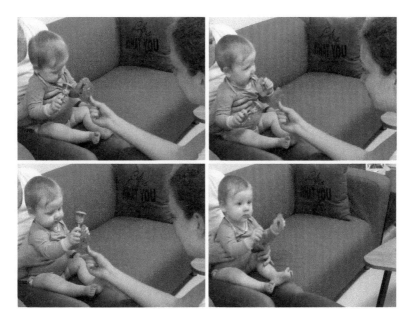

Figure 5.39 **Shows referential gazing (Item 61•)**

Item 52 Produces Strings of Syllables With Speech Melody – Also Assessed at 6 Months

POSITION

This item may be assessed in all positions (A).

PROCEDURE

During the assessment the assessor pays attention to the infant's vocalizations.

RECORDING

Typical performance means that the infant produces strings of syllables with speech melody (variation in pitch and volume), e.g. aionaba, wadabe, gedebe (Video 5.49).

Item 62• Identifies Desires With Gestures or Facial Expressions

POSITION

This item may be assessed in all positions (A).

PROCEDURE

During the assessment the assessor observes the infant's gestures and facial expressions.

RECORDING

Typical performance means that the infant identifies desires with gestures or facial expressions, with or without vocalizations. For instance, the infant moves their body towards the desired object, shakes their head, uses sustained gaze, repetitive vocalizations in combination with e.g. frowns and sulks (Video 5.59).

Item 63• Imitates Consonant–Vowel Sequences

POSITION

This item may be assessed in all positions (A).

PROCEDURE

The assessor or the parent engages in visual contact with the infant and addresses the infant with friendly strings of consonant–vowel sequences, such as gagaga, bababa, or doubidou. If the infant spontaneously addresses the adult with vocalizations, the assessor responds with their own series of consonant–vowel sequences. The assessor pays attention to the infant's vocalizations.

Recording

Typical performance means that the infant imitates the consonant–vowel sequences of the adult (Video 5.60).

Item 54   Visually Observes Falling and 'Crashing' Object – Also Assessed at 6 Months

Position

This item is assessed during supported sitting (Si).

Procedure

The assessor holds an attractive object in the infant's view and waits until the infant has visually explored the object. Next, the assessor drops the object, so that it clatters, i.e. 'crashes'. The assessor observes the infant's visual attention. If the infant does not respond to the first 'crash', the sequence is repeated once more.

Recording

Typical performance means that the infant visually follows the 'crashing' object to the floor (Fig. 5.33 and Video 5.51).

Item 64   Pays Visual Attention to Scribbling

Position

This item is assessed during sitting (Si).

Procedure

The assessor draws lines on a paper lying on a table in front of the infant. The assessor observes the infant's visual attention.

Recording

Typical performance means that the infant visually follows the assessor's hand movements or the pencil, or watches the emerging lines (Fig. 5.40 and Video 5.61).

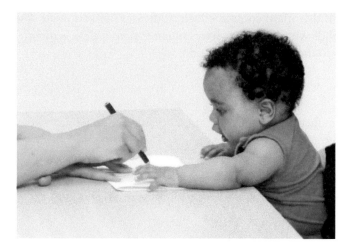

Figure 5.40 Pays visual attention to scribbling (Item 64)

Item 65   Produces Sound by Hitting With Object

POSITION

This item may be assessed in all positions (A).

PROCEDURE

The assessor offers the infant an attractive object, such as a ring, cube, or spoon, that, if hit on a surface (e.g. a table top), produces sound. The hitting should not be demonstrated. The assessor observes the infant's behaviour.

RECORDING

Typical performance means that the infant produces sound by hitting repeatedly with an object on a surface (Fig. 5.41 and Video 5.62).

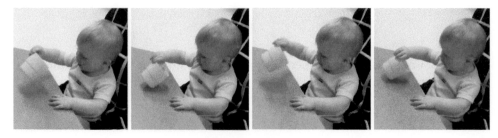

Figure 5.41 Produces sound by hitting with object (Item 65) The infant uses a plastic cup to make the sound.

Item 66   Grasps and Holds Two Objects for at Least 3 Seconds

POSITION

This item is assessed during sitting (Si).

PROCEDURE

The assessor presents an attractive object at reaching distance within the infant's visual field. When the infant has grasped the object, the assessor presents a second attractive object. The assessor observes the infant's arm and hand movements.

RECORDING

Typical performance means that the infant grasps and holds the first object. While holding the first object in their hand, they reach with the other hand towards the second object and grasp it. To pass the criterion, the infant needs to hold both objects for at least 3 seconds. The criterion is also passed when the infant uses only one hand for reaching, grasping, and holding the two objects (Fig. 5.42 and Video 5.63).

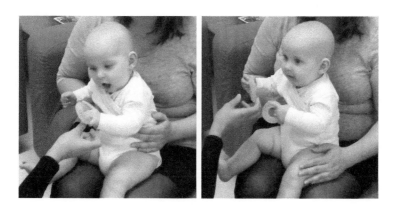

Figure 5.42 Grasps and holds two objects for at least 3 seconds (Item 66)

Item 67   Intentionally Pulls String to Obtain Object

POSITION

This item is assessed during sitting (Si).

PROCEDURE

Parent and infant sit on one side of a table. The assessor sits on the opposite side. The assessor has attached a string to an attractive object, such as a coloured ring, rattle, or a soft ball. The assessor moves the object to and fro by pulling the string until the infant

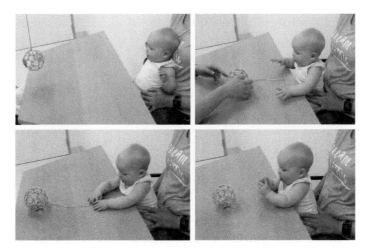

Figure 5.43 Intentionally pulls string to obtain object (Item 67)

pays sustained attention to the object. Next, they put the object out of reaching distance of the infant but the string within reaching distance, preferably at a right angle to the border of the table at which the parent and infant are sitting. The assessor tells the infant 'Get the object' (name of the object). They observe the infant's behaviour. If the infant does not respond, the sequence of events is repeated once more.

Recording

Typical performance means that the infant pulls the string to obtain the object and grasps the object (Fig. 5.43 and Video 5.64).

Item 68   Uses Scissor Grasp

Position

This item may be assessed in all positions (A).

Procedure

The assessor gives the infant a small, attractive object, such as a ring, a small animal, doll, or figure. The assessor observes the infant's finger movements.

Recording

Typical performance means that the infant grasps the object between extended thumb and extended index finger (Fig. 5.44).

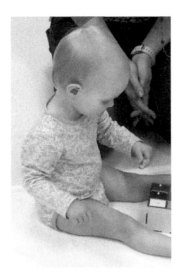

Figure 5.44 Uses scissor grasp (Item 68)

Item 69   Sits Independently for at Least 3 Seconds

POSITION

This item is assessed during sitting without support (Si).

PROCEDURE

The assessor puts the infant in sitting position on the assessment mattress while stabilizing the infant's trunk with their hands. They may put the infant's legs in semiflexion. Next, the assessor gradually withdraws their supporting hands. The assessor observes the infant's sitting behaviour. In infants who spontaneously adopt sitting position, spontaneous sitting behaviour is observed.

RECORDING

Typical performance means that the infant sits independently for at least 3 seconds, i.e. they are not supported by the assessor; the infant may use the support of their own hands (Video 5.65).

Item 70   Turns From Supine Into Prone

POSITION

This item is assessed in supine (Su).

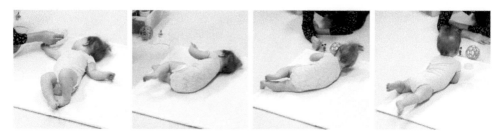

Figure 5.45 Turns from supine into prone (Item 70)

PROCEDURE

During the assessment the assessor observes whether the infant spontaneously turns from supine into prone position. If the infant does not show this behaviour spontaneously, the assessor presents an attractive object laterally within the upper visual field of the infant until the infant pays visual attention. Next, the assessor puts the object laterally to the infant, in such a way that it may elicit rolling behaviour. The assessor encourages the infant by saying 'Come on, get the object' (name of the object). The assessor observes the infant's motor behaviour.

RECORDING

Typical performance means that the infant turns from supine into prone position (Fig. 5.45 and Video 5.66).

Item 71   Reaches Out for Object in Prone

POSITION

This item is assessed in prone (P).

PROCEDURE

The assessor puts the infant in prone position with both shoulders in adduction and both elbows in flexion with the hands approximately in line with the ears. The prone position adopted by the infant after turning from supine may be an alternative starting position. The assessor puts an attractive object within the infant's lateral, upper visual field. They encourage the infant to get the object by saying 'Get the object' (name of the object). The assessor observes the infant's motor behaviour.

RECORDING

Typical performance means that the infant supports themself with one arm or hand and reaches with the other arm or hand in the direction of the object. To pass the criterion, the infant does not need to grasp the object (Fig. 5.46 and Video 5.67).

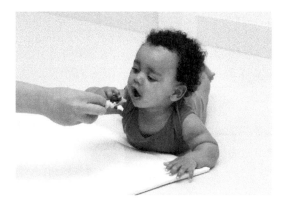

Figure 5.46 Reaches out for object in prone (Item 71)

Item 72   Pivots

POSITION

This item is assessed in prone (P).

PROCEDURE

The assessor puts the infant in prone position with both shoulders in slight adduction and both elbows in flexion with the hands approximately in line with the ears. The prone position adopted by the infant after turning from supine may be an alternative starting position. The assessor puts an attractive object within the infant's lateral visual field. They encourage the infant to get the object by saying 'Get the object' (name of the object). if the infant starts to move, the assessor gradually moves the object further laterally, so that the infant will pivot around its 'umbilical axis'. The assessor observes the infant's motor behaviour.

RECORDING

Typical performance means that the infant pivots around its 'umbilical axis' for at least 90° in prone position (Fig. 5.47 and Video 5.68).

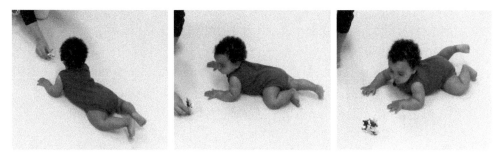

Figure 5.47 Pivots (Item 72)

DESCRIPTION OF THE DEVELOPMENTAL ITEMS TESTED AT 8 MONTHS

Item 60• Observes With Interest Peek-a-Boo Play – Also Assessed at 7 Months

POSITION

This item is assessed during sitting (Si).

PROCEDURE

In order to play peek-a-boo, the assessor engages in visual contact with the infant. Next, they 'hide' their face behind a sheet of paper or behind their hands, before uncovering themself after a few seconds, saying 'peek-a-boo!' If the infant does not respond, the procedure is repeated once more. The assessor observes the infant's behaviour.

RECORDING

Typical performance means that the infant shows interest in the peek-a-boo play by stopping other activities, directing visual attention to the assessor, changing facial expression, or vocalizing (Fig. 5.38 and Video 5.57).

Item 73• Imitates, e.g. Clapping of Hands or Waving When Encouraged

POSITION

This item is assessed during sitting (Si).

PROCEDURE

The assessor engages in visual contact with the infant. The assessor claps their hands, waves, or claps with their hands on the table. They playfully encourage the infant to join in and to imitate the movements shown. The assessor observes the infant's behaviour.

RECORDING

Typical performance means that the infant joins in and claps their hands, claps on the table, or waves (Video 5.69).

Item 52 Produces Strings of Syllables With Speech Melody – Also Assessed at 6 and 7 Months

POSITION

This item may be assessed in all positions (A).

Procedure

During the assessment the assessor pays attention to the infant's vocalizations.

Recording

Typical performance means that the infant produces strings of syllables with speech melody (variation in pitch and volume), e.g. aionaba, wadabe, gedebe (Video 5.49).

Item 62• Identifies Desires With Gestures or Facial Expressions – Also Assessed at 7 Months

Position

This item may be assessed in all positions (A).

Procedure

During the assessment the assessor observes the infant's gestures and facial expressions.

Recording

Typical performance means that the infant identifies desires with gestures or facial expressions, with or without vocalizations. For example, the infant moves their body towards the desired object, shakes their head, uses sustained gaze, repetitive vocalizations in combination with e.g. frowns and sulks (Video 5.59).

Item 63• Imitates Consonant–Vowel Sequences – Also Assessed at 7 Months

Position

This item may be assessed in all positions (A).

Procedure

The assessor or the parent engages in visual contact with the infant and addresses the infant with friendly strings of consonant–vowel sequences, such as gagaga, bababa, or doubidou. If the infant spontaneously addresses the adult with vocalizations, the assessor responds with their own series of consonant–vowel sequences. The assessor pays attention to the infant's vocalizations.

Recording

Typical performance means that the infant imitates the consonant–vowel sequences of the adult (Video 5.60).

Item 74•   Responds to Clear 'No'

POSITION

This item may be assessed in all positions (A).

PROCEDURE

The infant plays. The assessor or the parent utters a clear prohibitory 'no', either with or without associated gestures. The assessor observes the infant's behaviour.

RECORDING

Typical performance means that the infant's behaviour or facial expression changes, for instance stops behaviour or looks irritated (Video 5.70).

Item 64   Pays Visual Attention to Scribbling – Also Assessed at 7 Months

POSITION

This item is assessed during sitting (Si).

PROCEDURE

The assessor draws lines on a paper lying on a table in front of the infant. The assessor observes the infant's visual attention.

RECORDING

Typical performance means that the infant visually follows the assessor's hand movements or the pencil or watches the emerging lines (Fig. 5.40 and Video 5.61).

Item 75   Anticipatory Gaze to Object Reappearance

POSITION

This item is assessed during sitting (Si).

PROCEDURE

The assessor moves an attractive object to and fro within the infant's visual field behind a screen or a paper, showing it to the infant each time it peeps up at the edge of the screen or paper. Care is taken that the infant pays attention to the 'peeping up'. The

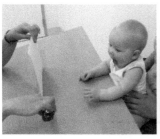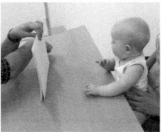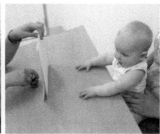

Figure 5.48 Anticipatory gaze to object reappearance (Item 75)

object is shown twice at each side. Next, the object disappears. The assessor observes the infant's visual attention.

RECORDING

Typical performance means that the infant observes the object and follows the moving object with their eyes, including when the object moves behind the screen or paper. The infant anticipates the 'peeping up' at the opposite edge of the screen or paper (Fig. 5.48 and Video 5.71).

Item 76   Looks at Pictures in Book

POSITION

This item is assessed during sitting (Si).

PROCEDURE

The assessor or parent shows the infant some pages of a baby book. The assessor or parent point to and name the pictures. The assessor observes the infant's visual attention.

RECORDING

Typical performance means that the infant pays attention to the pictures no less than two times for a duration of at least 2 seconds each time (Video 5.72).

Item 77   Turns Object to Explore it Visually

POSITION

This item may be assessed in all positions (A).

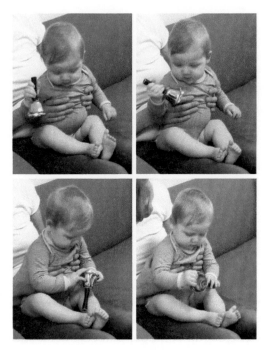

Figure 5.49 Turns object to explore it visually (Item 77)

PROCEDURE

The assessor gives the infant an attractive object with details, such as a small Mickey Mouse toy. The assessor observes the infant's visual attention and hand movements.

RECORDING

Typical performance means that the infant grasps the object, turns it around, and visually explores it (Fig. 5.49 and Video 5.73).

Item 67 Intentionally Pulls String to Obtain Object – Also Assessed at 7 Months

POSITION

This item is assessed during sitting (Si).

PROCEDURE

Parent and infant sit on one side of a table. The assessor sits on the opposite side. The assessor has attached a string to an attractive object, such as a coloured ring, rattle, or a soft ball. The assessor moves the object to and fro by pulling the string until the infant pays sustained attention to the object. Next, they put the object out of reaching distance of the infant but the string within reaching distance, preferably at a right angle to the border of the table at which the parent and infant are sitting. The assessor tells the infant 'Get the object' (name of the object). They observe the infant's behaviour. If the infant does not respond, the sequence of events is repeated once more.

RECORDING

Typical performance means that the infant pulls the string to obtain the object and grasps the object (Fig. 5.43 and Video 5.64).

Item 78   Tries to Pick Object From Cup

POSITION

This item is assessed during sitting (Si).

PROCEDURE

The assessor puts an attractive object, such as a coloured cube or a small puppet or figure, in a cup within the infant's visual field, within reaching distance. The assessor asks the infant to retrieve the object out of the cup by saying in a friendly way 'Did you see that? Can you get the object (name of object) out?' The assessor observes the infant's play behaviour.

RECORDING

Typical performance means that the infant tries to pick the object out of the cup with a hand (Fig. 5.50 and Video 5.74).

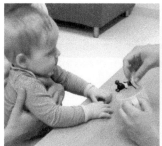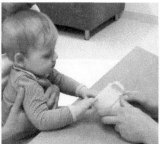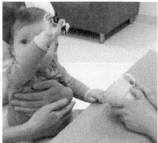

Figure 5.50 Tries to pick object from cup (Item 78)

Item 69   Sits Independently for at Least 3 Seconds – Also Assessed at 7 Months

POSITION

This item is assessed during sitting without support (Si).

PROCEDURE

The assessor puts the infant in sitting position on the assessment mattress while stabilizing the infant's trunk with their hands. They may put the infant's legs in semiflexion. Next, they gradually withdraw their supporting hands. The assessor observes the infant's sitting behaviour. In infants, who spontaneously adopt sitting position, spontaneous sitting behaviour is observed.

RECORDING

Typical performance means that the infant sits independently for at least 3 seconds, i.e. they are not supported by the assessor. The infant may use support of their own hands (Video 5.65).

Item 79   Gets On All Fours Independently

POSITION

This item is assessed during prone (P) or sitting (Si).

PROCEDURE

The infant is in prone position, is sitting on the floor, or moves down from a standing position. The assessor puts an attractive object within the infant's visual field but out of reach. The assessor encourages the infant to get the object by saying 'Get the object' (name of the object). The assessor observes the infant's motor behaviour.

RECORDING

Typical performance means that the infant moves from lying in prone, sitting, or squatting position into the 'all fours' position, i.e. in the prone posture, in which the body is supported by the knees (and lower legs) and hands. The abdomen does not touch the support surface. The infant does not need to move forward in the 'all fours' position (Fig. 5.51 and Video 5.75).

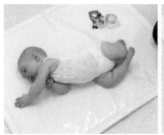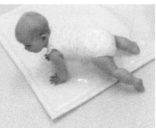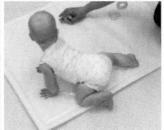

Figure 5.51 Gets on all fours independently (Item 79)

Item 80   Progression, e.g. Abdominal Crawling, Rolling

POSITION

This item is assessed during prone (P) or sitting (Si).

PROCEDURE

The infant is in prone or sitting position. The assessor puts an attractive object within the infant's visual field but out of reach. The assessor encourages the infant to get the object by saying 'Get the object' (name of the object). The assessor observes the infant's motor behaviour.

RECORDING

Typical performance means that the infant progresses through the room by abdominal crawling, rolling, or bottom shuffling. Progression may be either forwards, backwards, or laterally. Object retrieval is not a criterion to pass the item (Video 5.76).

DESCRIPTION OF THE DEVELOPMENTAL ITEMS TESTED AT 9 MONTHS

Item 73●   Imitates, e.g. Clapping of Hands or Waving When Encouraged – Also Assessed at 8 Months

POSITION

This item is assessed during sitting (Si).

PROCEDURE

The assessor engages in visual contact with the infant. The assessor claps their hands, waves, or claps with their hands on the table. They playfully encourage the infant to join in and to imitate the movements shown. The assessor observes the infant's behaviour.

RECORDING

Typical performance means that the infant joins in and claps their hands, claps on the table, or waves (Video 5.69).

Item 74●   Responds to Clear 'No' – Also Assessed at 8 Months

POSITION

This item may be assessed in all positions (A).

Procedure

The infant plays. The assessor or the parent utters a clear prohibitory 'no', either with or without associated gestures. The assessor observes the infant's behaviour.

Recording

Typical performance means that the infant's behaviour or facial expression changes, for instance stops behaviour or looks irritated (Video 5.70).

Item 81   Produces Chains of Three Syllables (Canonical Babbling)

Position

This item may be assessed in all positions (A).

Procedure

During the assessment the assessor pays attention to the infant's vocalizations. The vocalizations may occur spontaneously or when being talked to by the assessor or parent.

Recording

Typical performance means that the infant produces chains of three identical syllables (canonical babbling), e.g. da-da-da, ma-ma-ma, or be-be-be (Video 5.77).

Item 82•   Responds to Own Name

Position

This item may be assessed in all positions (A).

Procedure

The assessor asks the parent by which name the infant is usually called. When the infant is playing during the assessment, the assessor calls the infant by their name. After a few seconds they call the infant by using a simple word that is generally unknown to infants, such as 'camel'. If the infant does not clearly respond at the first trial with their own name and the unknown word or the difference between the two calls is not clear, the sequence of the two calls (the infant's name and the unknown word) is repeated two additional times. The assessor observes the infant's behaviour.

Recording

Typical performance means that the infant clearly responds when their own name is mentioned, but they do not show a similar reaction to the unknown word (Video 5.78).

Item 75 Anticipatory Gaze to Object Reappearance – Also Assessed at 8 Months

POSITION

This item is assessed during sitting (Si).

PROCEDURE

The assessor moves an attractive object to and fro behind a screen or a paper within the visual field, showing it to the infant each time it peeps up at the edge of the screen or paper. Care is taken that the infant pays attention to the 'peeping up'. The object is shown twice at each side. Next, the object disappears. The assessor observes the infant's visual attention.

RECORDING

Typical performance means that the infant observes the object and follows the moving object with their eyes, including when the object moves behind the screen or paper. The infant anticipates the 'peeping up' at the opposite edge of the screen or paper (Fig. 5.48 and Video 5.71).

Item 76 Looks at Pictures in Book – Also Assessed at 8 Months

POSITION

This item is assessed during sitting (Si).

PROCEDURE

The assessor or parent shows the infant some pages of a baby book. They point to and name the pictures. The assessor observes the infant's visual attention.

RECORDING

Typical performance means that the infant looks at the pictures no less than two times for a duration of at least 2 seconds each time (Video 5.72).

Item 83 Intentionally Rings Bell

POSITION

This item is assessed during sitting (Si).

PROCEDURE

The assessor shows the infant the bell. They ring the bell and give it to the infant. The assessor observes the infant's behaviour.

RECORDING

Typical performance means that the infant intentionally rings the bell. Intentional ringing of the bell does not include hitting table with the bell (Video 5.79).

Item 67   Intentionally Pulls String to Obtain Object – Also Assessed at 7 and 8 Months

POSITION

This item is assessed during sitting (Si).

PROCEDURE

The parent and infant sit on one side of a table. The assessor sits on the opposite side. The assessor has attached a string to an attractive object, such as a coloured ring, rattle, or a soft ball. The assessor moves the object to and fro by pulling the string until the infant pays sustained attention to the object. Next, they put the object out of reaching distance of the infant but the string within reaching distance, preferably at a right angle to the border of the table at which the parent and infant are sitting. The assessor tells the infant 'Get the object' (name of the object). They observe the infant's behaviour. If the infant does not respond, the sequence of events is repeated once more.

RECORDING

Typical performance means that the infant pulls the string to obtain the object and grasps the object (Fig. 5.43 and Video 5.64).

Item 84   Removes Obstacle to Get Object

POSITION

This item is assessed during sitting (Si).

PROCEDURE

The assessor shows the infant an attractive object. They emphasize this by saying, 'Look, this is nice' (or something similar). They put the object on the table in front of the infant. Next, they put a roll of neutral cloth (e.g. a cloth diaper) as an obstacle between the object and the infant, in such a way that the infant has to remove the cloth in order to retrieve the object. The cloth itself should not be attractive. The assessor observes the infant's behaviour.

RECORDING

Typical performance means that the infant removes the cloth and grasps the object (Fig. 5.52 and Video 5.80).

Atypical performance means that the infant does not meet the criteria for typical performance, for example the infant grasps the cloth and plays with the cloth or the infant turns away.

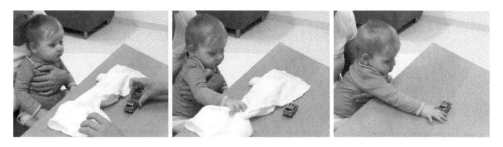

Figure 5.52 **Removes obstacle to get object (Item 84)**

Item 85 Explores Details of Object With Fingertips

Position

This item is assessed during sitting (Si).

Procedure

The assessor gives the infant an attractive object with details, such as a small Mickey Mouse toy. The assessor observes the infant's visual attention and hand and finger movements.

Recording

Typical performance means that the infant explores the object, turns it around, inspects it from various sides, and uses the fingertips for exploration. The infant may also put the object temporarily in their mouth (Fig. 5.53 and Video 5.81).

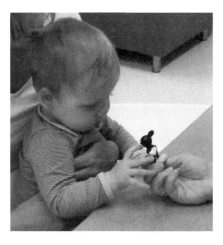

Figure 5.53 **Explores details of object with fingertips (Item 85)**

Item 86   Puts Object In Cup

POSITION

This item is assessed during sitting (Si).

PROCEDURE

The assessor puts a cup on the table in front of the infant. The assessor puts a small object in the cup and retrieves it again. Next, the assessor hands the object to the infant, puts the cup on the table in front of the infant, and tells the infant to do the same by saying 'Can you do the same? Can you put the object (name of the object) in the cup?' The assessor repeats the demonstration once again. Then it is the infant's turn. The infant is offered some time. The assessor observes the infant's behaviour.

RECORDING

Typical performance means that the infant puts the object in the cup (Fig. 5.54 and Video 5.82).

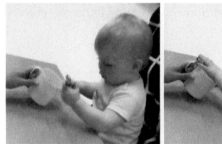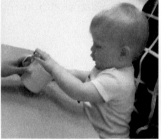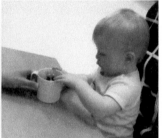

Figure 5.54 Puts object in cup (Item 86)

Item 87   Sits Independently for Sustained Periods of Time

POSITION

This item is assessed during sitting without support (Si).

PROCEDURE

The assessor puts the infant in sitting position on the assessment mattress while stabilizing the infant's trunk with their hands. Next, they gradually withdraw their supporting hands. The assessor observes the infant's sitting behaviour. In infants who spontaneously adopt sitting position, spontaneous sitting behaviour is observed.

Typical performance means that the infant sits independently for a sustained period of time (at least half a minute) without support. W-sitting, i.e. sitting between the knees with the legs in W-form is also considered as a form of independent sitting. Support of the hands is not allowed (Video 5.83).

Item 88   Sits Independently and Rotates Trunk

POSITION

This item is assessed during sitting without support (Si).

PROCEDURE

The assessor puts the infant in sitting position on the assessment mattress while stabilizing the infant's trunk with their hands. Next, they gradually withdraw their supporting hands. The infant may also move themself into sitting position. The assessor shows the infant an attractive object and moves the object laterally a bit beyond the infant's bottom. Rotation to both sides is tested. The assessor observes the infant's sitting behaviour.

RECORDING

Typical performance means that the infant sits independently and is able to rotate the trunk on at least one side for more than 30° (Fig. 5.55 and Video 5.84).

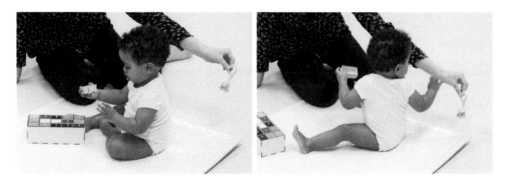

Figure 5.55 Sits independently and rotates trunk (Item 88)

Item 89   Stands on Knees While Holding on to Furniture

POSITION

This item may be assessed from all starting positions (A).

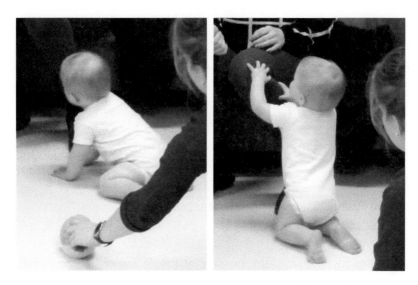

Figure 5.56 Stands on knees while holding on to furniture (Item 89) Note that not only furniture may be used, but also parental legs. Yet, the parent should not pull the infant up.

Procedure

The assessor or the parent puts an attractive object on a stool or similar piece of furniture and encourages the infant to get the object. The assessor observes the infant's motor behaviour.

Recording

Typical performance means that the infant pulls themself to the knee standing position while holding on to a stool or other piece of furniture (Fig. 5.56 and Video 5.85).

Item 90   Progression On All Fours, Bunny Hop, Bottom Shuffling

Position

This item is assessed during prone (P) or sitting (Si).

Procedure

The assessor puts an attractive object on the floor, out of the infant's reach. They encourage the infant to get the object. The assessor observes the infant's motor behaviour.

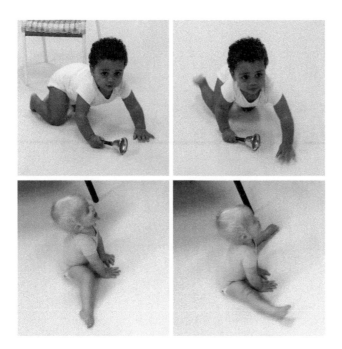

Figure 5.57 Progression on all fours, bunny hop, bottom shuffling (Item 90) Upper panel: progression on all fours, lower panel: bottom shuffling.

RECORDING

Typical performance means that the infant moves forward by crawling on all fours, bunny hopping, or bottom shuffling. During progression the abdomen does not touch the support surface (Fig. 5.57 and Video 5.86).

DESCRIPTION OF THE DEVELOPMENTAL ITEMS TESTED AT 10 MONTHS

Item 91• Imitates Play of 'Clap Your Hands' or Other Hand or Finger Play

POSITION

This item is assessed during sitting (Si).

PROCEDURE

The assessor demonstrates within the infant's view the 'clap your hands' song and play or similar infant rhymes with accompanying hand or finger play. They encourage the infant to join in. The assessor observes the infant's motor behaviour.

Recording

Typical performance means that the infant imitates the 'clap your hands' or the other hand or finger play (Video 5.87).

Item 92• Uses Different Expressions or Gestures for Known and Unknown Persons

Position

This item may be assessed in all positions (A).

Procedure

During the assessment the assessor pays attention to the infant's interactions with other persons.

Recording

Typical performance means that the infant's facial expressions or gestures in interaction with known persons differ from those used in interaction with unknown persons (Video 5.88).

Item 82• Responds to Own Name – Also Assessed at 9 Months

Position

This item may be assessed in all positions (A).

Procedure

The assessor asks the parent by which name the infant is usually called. When the infant is playing during the assessment the assessor calls the infant by their name. After a few seconds they call the infant by using a simple word that is generally unknown to infants, such as 'camel'. If the infant does not clearly respond at the first trial with their own name and the unknown word, or the difference between the two calls is not clear, the sequence of the two calls (the infant's name and the unknown word) is repeated two additional times. The assessor observes the infant's behaviour.

Recording

Typical performance means that the infant clearly responds when their own name is mentioned but they do not show a similar reaction to the unknown word (Video 5.78).

Item 93• Responds to Question: 'Where is ...?' (Object, Person)

Position

This item may be assessed in all positions (A).

PROCEDURE

The assessor shows the infant an attractive and known object A and puts it on the table (check with parent which objects the infant knows). Next, the assessor shows the infant another attractive object B and asks 'Where is object A?' If this question does not result in an adequate response, the assessor may ask 'Where is mama?' (or other well-known person who is around). The assessor observes the infant's behaviour.

RECORDING

Typical performance means that the infant directs visual attention, the hand or fingers, or the entire body to object A or a well-known person, respectively (Video 5.89).

Item 94   Produces at Least Two Different Chains of Three Syllables

POSITION

This item may be assessed in all positions (A).

PROCEDURE

During the assessment the assessor pays attention to the infant's vocalizations. The vocalizations may occur spontaneously and when being talked to by the assessor or parent.

RECORDING

Typical performance means that the infant produces at least two different chains of three identical syllables (canonical babbling), e.g. da-da-da, ma-ma-ma, or be-be-be (Video 5.90).

Item 83   Intentionally Rings Bell – Also Assessed at 9 Months

POSITION

This item is assessed during sitting (Si).

PROCEDURE

The assessor shows the infant the bell. The assessor rings the bell and gives it to the infant. The assessor observes the infant's behaviour.

RECORDING

Typical performance means that the infant intentionally rings the bell. Intentional ringing of the bell does not include hitting the table with a bell (Video 5.79).

Item 95   Looks at Pictures in Book and Turns Pages

POSITION

This item is assessed during sitting (Si).

PROCEDURE

The assessor or parent shows the infant some pages of a baby book. The assessor points to and names the pictures and turns pages. Next, they encourage the infant to turn the next page: 'And, now you, it is your turn'. The assessor observes the infant's behaviour.

RECORDING

Typical performance means that the infant pays attention to the pictures shown and turns a page no less than two times, with the infant paying attention to the pictures for at least 2 seconds each time (Fig. 5.58 and Video 5.91).

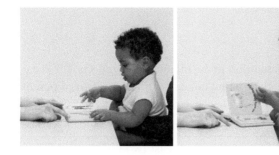 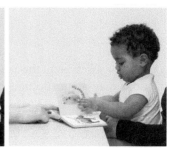

Figure 5.58 **Looks at pictures in book and turns pages (Item 95)**

Item 96•   Engages in Joint Exploration (Joint Attention)

POSITION

This item may be assessed in all positions (A).

PROCEDURE

The parent is instructed to perform the following sequence of actions: to engage in visual contact with the infant, to point to an attractive object, to look to the infant, and to say to the infant: 'Look!' The assessor observes the infant's behaviour.

RECORDING

Typical performance means that the infant looks to the parent in the joint exploration of the object (Fig. 5.59 and Video 5.92).

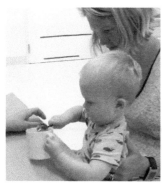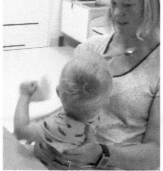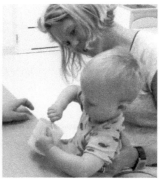

Figure 5.59 Engages in joint exploration (joint attention) (Item 96•)

Item 85   Explores Details of Object With Fingertips – Also Assessed at 9 Months

POSITION

This item is assessed during sitting (Si).

PROCEDURE

The assessor gives the infant an attractive object with details, such as a small Mickey Mouse toy. The assessor observes the infant's visual attention and hand and finger movements.

RECORDING

Typical performance means that the infant explores the object, turns it around, inspects it from various sides, and uses the fingertips for exploration. The infant may also put the object temporarily in their mouth (Fig. 5.53 and Video 5.81).

Item 86   Puts Object In Cup – Also Assessed at 9 Months

POSITION

This item is assessed during sitting (Si).

PROCEDURE

The assessor puts a cup on the table in front of the infant. The assessor puts a small object in the cup and retrieves it again. Next, they hand the object to the infant, put the cup on the table in front of the infant, and tell the infant to do the same by saying 'Can you do the same? Can you put the object (name of the object) in the cup?' The assessor repeats the demonstration once again. Then it is the infant's turn. The infant is offered some time. The assessor observes the infant's behaviour.

RECORDING

Typical performance means that the infant puts the object in the cup (Fig. 5.54 and Video 5.82).

Item 97   Uses Index Finger to Touch Details of Object

POSITION

This item may be assessed in all positions (A).

PROCEDURE

The assessor gives the infant an attractive object with details, such as a small Mickey Mouse toy. The assessor observes the infant's finger movements.

RECORDING

Typical performance means that the infant uses their index finger to touch the details of the object (Fig. 5.60 and Video 5.93).

Atypical performance means that the infant does not meet the criteria for typical performance, e.g. the infant uses the tips of multiple fingers simultaneously to touch the details of the object.

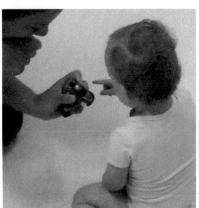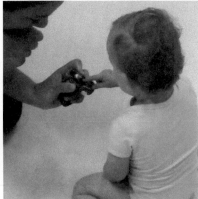

Figure 5.60 Infant aged 9 months uses their index finger to touch details of object (Item 97)

Item 88   Sits Independently and Rotates Trunk – Also Assessed
at 9 Months

POSITION

This item is assessed during sitting without support (Si).

PROCEDURE

The assessor puts the infant in sitting position on the assessment mattress while stabilizing the infant's trunk with their hands. Next, they gradually withdraw their supporting hands, or the infant moves themself into sitting position. The assessor shows the infant an attractive object and moves the object laterally a bit beyond the infant's bottom. Rotation to both sides is tested. The assessor observes the infant's sitting behaviour.

Recording

Typical performance means that the infant sits independently and is able to rotate the trunk on at least one side for more than 30° (Fig. 5.55 and Video 5.84).

Item 90   Progression On All Fours, Bunny Hop, Bottom Shuffling – Also Assessed at 9 Months

Position

This item is assessed during prone (P) or sitting (Si).

Procedure

The assessor puts an attractive object on the floor, out of the infant's reach. They encourage the infant to get the object. The assessor observes the infant's motor behaviour.

Recording

Typical performance means that the infant moves forward by crawling on all fours, bunny hopping, or bottom shuffling. During progression the abdomen does not touch the support surface (Fig. 5.57 and Video 5.86).

Item 98   Gets Into Sitting Position Independently

Position

This item is assessed from supine (Su) or prone (P) starting positions.

Procedure

The infant moves themself from supine or prone position into sitting position. If the infant does not move themself into sitting position, the assessor presents the infant an attractive object in such a way that the infant may move into sitting position.

Recording

Typical performance means that the infant gets into sitting position independently and is able to maintain a sitting position (see Item 87). W-sitting, i.e. sitting between the knees with the legs in W-form, is also considered as a form of independent sitting (Video 5.94).

Item 99   Pulls to Stand

POSITION

This item may be assessed from all starting positions (A).

PROCEDURE

The assessor or the parent puts an attractive object on a stool or other relatively low piece of furniture, and they encourage the infant to get the object. The assessor observes the infant's motor behaviour.

RECORDING

Typical performance means that the infant pulls themself into standing position with the help of the furniture or the legs of the parent (without further assistance) (Fig. 5.61 and Video 5.95).

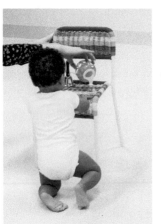 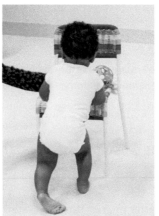 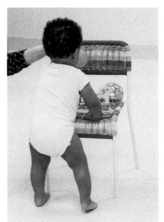

Figure 5.61 Pulls to stand (Item 99)

DESCRIPTION OF THE DEVELOPMENTAL ITEMS TESTED AT 11 MONTHS

Item 91•   Imitates Play of 'Clap Your Hands' or Other Hand or Finger Play – Also Assessed at 10 Months

POSITION

This item is assessed during sitting (Si).

PROCEDURE

The assessor demonstrates within the infant's view the 'clap your hands' song and play, or similar infant rhymes with accompanying hand or finger play. They encourage the infant to join in. The assessor observes the infant's motor behaviour.

RECORDING

Typical performance means that the infant imitates the 'clap your hands' or the other hand or finger play (Video 5.87).

Item 82• Responds to Own Name – Also Assessed at 9 and 10 Months

POSITION

This item may be assessed in all positions (A).

PROCEDURE

The assessor asks the parent by which name the infant is usually called. When the infant is playing during the assessment the assessor calls the infant by their name. After a few seconds they call the infant by using a simple word that is generally unknown to infants, such as 'camel'. If the infant does not clearly respond at the first trial with their own name and the unknown word, or the difference between the two calls is not clear, the sequence of the two calls (the infant's name and the unknown word) is repeated two additional times. The assessor observes the infant's behaviour.

RECORDING

Typical performance means that the infant clearly responds when their own name is mentioned, but they do not show a similar reaction to the unknown word (Video 5.78).

Item 93• Responds to Question: 'Where is …?' (Object, Person) – Also Assessed at 10 Months

POSITION

This item may be assessed in all positions (A).

PROCEDURE

The assessor shows the infant an attractive and known object A and puts it on the table (check with parent which objects the infant knows). Next, the assessor shows the infant another attractive object B and asks 'Where is object A?' If this question does not result in an adequate response, the assessor may ask 'Where is mama?' (or other well-known person who is around). The assessor observes the infant's behaviour.

Recording

Typical performance means that the infant directs visual attention, the hand or fingers, or the entire body to object A or the well-known person, respectively (Video 5.89).

Item 94   Produces at Least Two Different Chains of Three Syllables – Also Assessed at 10 Months

Position

This item may be assessed in all positions (A).

Procedure

During the assessment the assessor pays attention to the infant's vocalizations. The vocalizations may occur spontaneously and when being talked to by the assessor or parent.

Recording

Typical performance means that the infant produces at least two different chains of three identical syllables (canonical babbling), e.g. da-da-da, ma-ma-ma, or be-be-be (Video 5.90).

Item 83   Intentionally Rings Bell – Also Assessed at 9 and 10 Months

Position

This item is assessed during sitting (Si).

Procedure

The assessor shows the infant the bell. They ring the bell and give it to the infant. The assessor observes the infant's behaviour.

Recording

Typical performance means that the infant intentionally rings the bell. Intentional ringing of the bell does not include hitting the table with the bell (Video 5.79).

Item 95   Looks at Pictures in Book and Turns Pages – Also Assessed at 10 Months

Position

This item is assessed during sitting (Si).

PROCEDURE

The assessor or parent shows the infant some pages of a baby book. They point to and name the pictures, and they turn pages. Next, they encourage the infant to turn the next page: 'And, now you, it is your turn.' The assessor observes the infant's behaviour.

RECORDING

Typical performance means that the infant pays attention to the pictures shown and turns a page no less than two times, with the infant paying attention to the pictures for at least 2 seconds each time (Fig. 5.58 and Video 5.91).

Item 96● Engages in Joint Exploration (Joint Attention) – Also Assessed at 10 Months

POSITION

This item may be assessed in all positions (A).

PROCEDURE

The parent is instructed to perform the following sequence of actions: to engage in visual contact with the infant, to point to an attractive object, to look to the infant, and to say to the infant: 'Look!' The assessor observes the infant's behaviour.

RECORDING

Typical performance means that the infant looks to the parent in the joint exploration of the object (Fig. 5.59 and Video 5.92).

Item 100 Finds Object Covered by Cup

POSITION

This item is assessed during sitting (Si).

PROCEDURE

The assessor shows the infant an attractive object and a cup. They offer them to the infant to play with. Next, the assessor hides the object in front of the infant by covering it with the cup. They ask t he infant: 'Where is the object (name of the object)? Can you get it?' The assessor observes the infant's behaviour.

RECORDING

Typical performance means that the infant lifts the cup and discovers the object (Fig. 5.62 and Video 5.96).

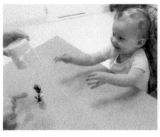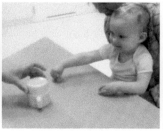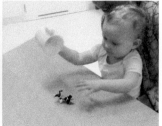

Figure 5.62 Finds object covered by cup (Item 100)

Item 97 Uses Index Finger to Touch Details of Object – Also Assessed at 10 Months

POSITION

This item may be assessed in all positions (A).

PROCEDURE

The assessor gives the infant an attractive object with details, such as a small Mickey Mouse toy. The assessor observes the infant's finger movements.

RECORDING

Typical performance means that the infant uses their index finger to touch the details of the object (Fig. 5.60 and Video 5.93).

Atypical performance means that the infant does not meet the criteria for typical performance, for example the infant uses the tips of multiple fingers simultaneously to touch the details of the object.

Item 101 Holds Two Objects and Grasps Third Object

POSITION

This item is assessed during sitting (Si).

PROCEDURE

The assessor presents attractive objects, such as rings, small puppets, animals, and figures to the infant. If the infant is able to hold two objects, the assessor presents a third attractive object, and they encourage the infant to grasp it. The assessor observes the infant's motor behaviour.

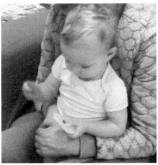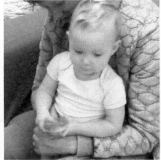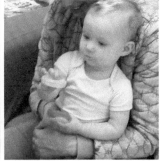

Figure 5.63 Holds two objects and grasps third object (Item 101)

Recording

Typical performance means that the infant grasps the third object, while holding the other two objects as well. The infant's body may serve as a supportive device, i.e. one of the held objects may be clamped between arm and body (Fig. 5.63 and Video 5.97).

Item 102   Uses Spoon to Stir In Cup or On Plate (in Imitation)

Position

This item is assessed during sitting (Si).

Procedure

The assessor shows the infant a spoon and a cup or plate. They show the infant how to stir with the spoon in the cup or on the plate. They encourage the infant to do the same. The assessor observes the infant's behaviour.

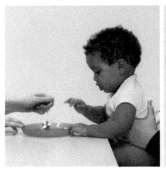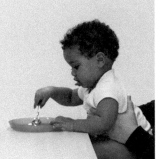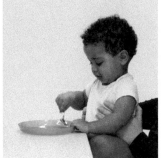

Figure 5.64 Uses spoon to stir in cup or on plate (in imitation) (Item 102)

Typical performance means that the infant produces circular or to and fro movements to stir with the spoon in the cup or on the plate (Fig. 5.64 and Video 5.98).

Item 103 Pulls the Right String to Retrieve Object

POSITION

This item is assessed during sitting (Si).

PROCEDURE

The parent and infant sit on one side of a table. The assessor sits on the opposite side. The assessor has attached a coloured string to an attractive object, such as a coloured ring, rattle, or a soft ball. They put the object on the table out of the infant's reach. They stretch the string out on the table in the direction of the infant, with the end of the string within reaching distance. Next, the assessor shows a second coloured string (similar to the first string) without an object. They put the second string in parallel with the first one, the distance between the two strings being about 15cm. The assessor encourages the infant to retrieve the object: 'Get the object (name of the object)'. If the first trial is not successful, a second trial, in which the whole sequence of events is repeated, may be attempted. The assessor observes the infant's behaviour.

RECORDING

Typical performance means that the infant grasps the string that is connected to the object, and pulls it so that the object moves in the infant's direction (Fig. 5.65 and Video 5.99).

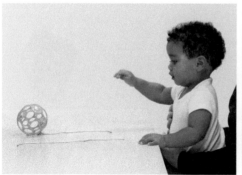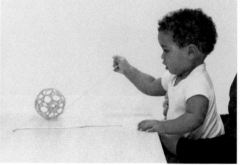

Figure 5.65 Pulls the right string to retrieve object (Item 103)

Item 90   Progression On All Fours, Bunny Hop, Bottom Shuffling –
Also Assessed at 9 and 10 Months

POSITION

This item is assessed during prone (P) or sitting (Si).

PROCEDURE

The assessor puts an attractive object on the floor, out of the infant's reach. They encourage the infant to get the object. The assessor observes the infant's motor behaviour.

RECORDING

Typical performance means that the infant moves forward by crawling on all fours, bunny hopping, or bottom shuffling. During progression the abdomen does not touch the support surface (Fig. 5.57 and Video 5.86).

Item 99   Pulls to Stand – Also Assessed at 10 Months

POSITION

This item may be assessed from all starting positions (A).

PROCEDURE

The assessor or the parent puts an attractive object on a stool or other relatively low piece of furniture, and encourages the infant to get the object.

RECORDING

Typical performance means that the infant pulls themself with the help of the furniture or the legs of the parent (without further assistance) into standing position (Fig. 5.61 and Video 5.95).

Item 104   Cruises Along Furniture

POSITION

This item is assessed during standing (St).

PROCEDURE

The assessor puts an attractive object on a stool, a chair, or other piece of relatively low furniture, and encourages the infant to get the object. Next, the object is moved, so that the infant is challenged to cruise along the furniture. The assessor observes the infant's motor behaviour.

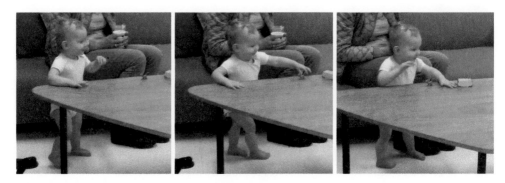

Figure 5.66 Cruises along furniture (Item 104)

Recording

Typical performance means that the infant cruises with at least three steps along the furniture (Fig. 5.66 and Video 5.100).

DESCRIPTION OF THE DEVELOPMENTAL ITEMS TESTED AT 12 MONTHS

Item 93• Responds to Question: 'Where is ...?' (Object, Person) – Also Assessed at 10 and 11 Months

Position

This item may be assessed in all positions (A).

Procedure

The assessor shows the infant an attractive and known object A and puts it on the table (check with parent which objects the infant knows). Next, the assessor shows the infant another attractive object B and asks 'Where is object A?' If this question does not result in an adequate response, the assessor may ask 'Where is mama?' (or other well-known person who is around). The assessor observes the infant's behaviour.

Recording

Typical performance means that the infant directs visual attention, the hand or fingers, or the entire body to object A or well-known person, respectively (Video 5.89).

Item 105• Shows Semantic Gestures When Challenged

Position

This item may be assessed in all positions (A).

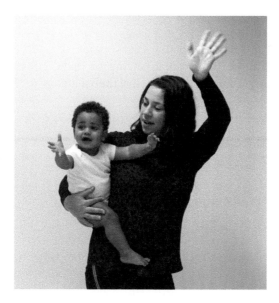

Figure 5.67 Shows semantic gestures when challenged (Item 105)

PROCEDURE

During the assessment the assessor pays attention to the presence of semantic gestures, such as 'pointing (with index finger, hand, or arm)', 'bye-bye' (spontaneously when leaving the assessment room), or 'shaking of the head'. If the infant has not shown the gestures during the course of the assessment, the assessor may ask the infant 'Where is mama?', 'Where is the car?' 'Show me the bear' etc. Note that the gestures should not be demonstrated.

RECORDING

Typical performance means that the infant independently shows semantic gestures (Fig. 5.67 and Video 5.101).

Item 106• Uses 'Mama' Or 'Dada' or Other Meaningful Word

POSITION

This item may be assessed in all positions (A).

PROCEDURE

During the assessment the assessor pays attention to the vocalizations of the infant.

RECORDING

Typical performance means that the infant uses 'mama' or 'dada' for the correct person, or uses one meaningful word other than 'mama' or 'dada'. The meaningful word does not need to be pronounced perfectly, i.e. 'na-na' for banana or 'da' for dog (Video 5.102).

Item 95   Looks at Pictures in Book and Turns Pages –
Also Assessed at 10 and 11 Months

POSITION

This item is assessed during sitting (Si).

PROCEDURE

The assessor or parent shows the infant some pages of a baby book. They point to and name the pictures, and they turn pages. Next, they encourage the infant to turn the next page: 'And, now you. It is your turn.' The assessor observes the infant's behaviour.

RECORDING

Typical performance means that the infant pays attention to the pictures shown and turns a page no less than two times, with the infant paying attention to the pictures for at least 2 seconds each time (Video 5.91).

Item 96•   Engages in Joint Exploration (Joint Attention) – Also Assessed
at 10 and 11 Months

POSITION

This item may be assessed in all positions (A).

PROCEDURE

The parent is instructed to perform the following sequence of actions: to engage in visual contact with the infant, to point to an attractive object, to look to the infant, and to say to the infant: 'Look!' The assessor observes the infant's behaviour.

RECORDING

Typical performance means that the infant looks to the parent in the joint exploration of the object (Fig. 5.59 and Video 5.92).

Item 107   Finds Object Hidden Under One of Two Cups

POSITION

This item is assessed during sitting (Si).

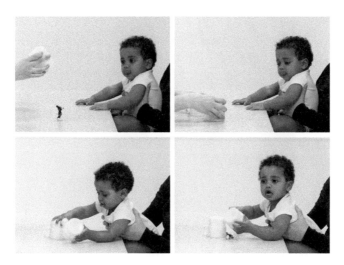

Figure 5.68 Finds object hidden under one of two cups (Item 107)

PROCEDURE

The assessor shows the infant an attractive object and two cups. They offer the material to the infant to play with. Next, the assessor hides the object in front of the infant by covering it with one of the cups. They ask the infant: 'Where is the object (name of the object)? Can you get it?' The assessor observes the infant's behaviour.

RECORDING

Typical performance means that the infant looks to the right cup, lifts it, and discovers the object (Fig. 5.68 and Video 5.103).

Item 108● Points With Index Finger to Persons or Objects

POSITION

This item may be assessed in all positions (A).

PROCEDURE

During the assessment the assessor observes the infant's behaviour. The infant may point spontaneously or in response to question 'Where is … (person, object)?'.

RECORDING

Typical performance means that the infant points with their index finger to an object or a person (Fig. 5.69 and Video 5.104).

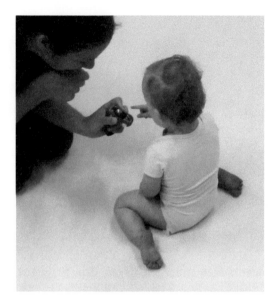

Figure 5.69 Points with index finger to persons or objects (Item 108•)

Item 101   Holds Two Objects and Grasps Third Object – Also Assessed at 11 Months

POSITION

This item is assessed during sitting (Si).

PROCEDURE

The assessor presents attractive objects, such as rings, small puppets, animals, and figures to the infant. If the infant is able to hold two objects, the assessor presents a third attractive object, and they encourage the infant to grasp it. The assessor observes the infant's motor behaviour.

RECORDING

Typical performance means that the infant grasps the third object, while holding the other two objects as well. The infant's body may serve as a supportive device, i.e. one of the held objects may be clamped between arm and body (Fig. 5.63 and Video 5.97).

Item 102   Uses Spoon to Stir In Cup or On Plate (in Imitation) – Also Assessed at 11 Months

POSITION

This item is assessed during sitting (Si).

Procedure

The assessor shows the infant a spoon and a cup or plate. They show the infant how to stir with the spoon in the cup or on the plate. They encourage the infant to do the same. The assessor observes the infant's behaviour.

Recording

Typical performance means that the infant produces circular or to and fro movements to stir with the spoon in the cup or on the plate (Fig. 5.64 and Video 5.98).

Item 103   Pulls the Right String to Retrieve Object – Also Assessed at 11 Months

Position

This item is assessed during sitting (Si).

Procedure

Parent and infant are sitting on one side of a table. The assessor sits on the opposite side. The assessor has attached a coloured string to an attractive object, such as a coloured ring, rattle, or a soft ball. They put the object on the table out of the infant's reach. They stretch the string out on the table in the direction of the infant, with the end of the string within reaching distance. Next, the assessor shows a second coloured string (similar to the first string) without an object. They put the second string in parallel with the first one, the distance between the two strings being about 15cm. The assessor encourages the infant to retrieve the object: 'Get the object (name of the object)'. If the first trial is not successful, a second trial, in which the whole sequence of events is repeated, may be attempted. The assessor observes the infant's behaviour.

Recording

Typical performance means that the infant grasps the string that is connected to the object and pulls it so that the object moves in the infant's direction (Fig. 5.65 and Video 5.99).

Item 109   Uses Pincer Grasp

Position

This item may be assessed in all positions (A).

Procedure

The assessor presents the infant a small attractive object, such as a narrow measuring tape, a string, a breadcrumb, and a raisin, and they encourage the infant to grasp it. The assessor observes the infant's hand and finger movements. Please take care when presenting small non-edible objects that the infant does not swallow them.

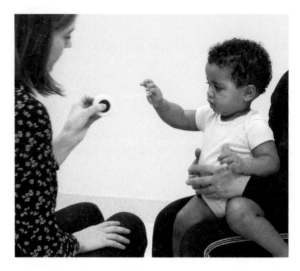

Figure 5.70 Uses pincer grasp (Item 109) Note: a retractable measurement tape with a case works very well to elicit a pincer grasp.

RECORDING

Typical performance means that the infant uses the pincer grasp, i.e. they grasp the object between the tips of the thumb and the index finger. The third finger may be close to the two grasping fingers but should not be involved in the actual task of the precision grip (Fig. 5.70 and Video 5.105).

Item 110   Throws Small Ball Forward

POSITION

This item is assessed during sitting (Si).

PROCEDURE

The assessor or the parent gives the infant a small ball (or another object) in the hand. They encourage the infant to throw the ball (or object) in their direction. When the infant does not respond with throwing, the action of throwing is demonstrated: either the assessor or the parent throw the ball to the infant, or the assessor throws the ball to the parent. The assessor observes the behaviour of the infant.

RECORDING

Typical performance means that the infant throws the ball (or object) forward (Fig. 5.71 and Video 5.106).

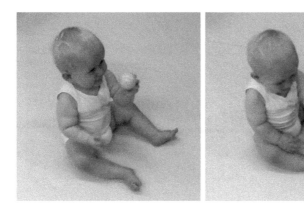

Figure 5.71 Throws small ball forward (Item 110)

Item 111   Stands Independently for at Least 3 Seconds

POSITION

This item is assessed during standing (St).

PROCEDURE

The assessor or the parent supports the standing infant by holding one hand. Next, hand support is gradually withdrawn so that the infant stands independently. The assessor observes the motor behaviour of the infant.

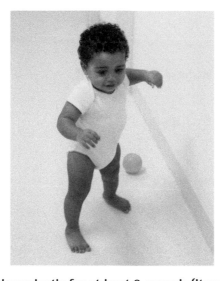

Figure 5.72 Stands independently for at least 3 seconds (Item 111)

Typical performance means that the infant stands independently for at least 3 seconds (Fig. 5.72 and Video 5.107).

Item 112   Walks When One Hand Held

POSITION

This item is assessed during standing (St).

PROCEDURE

The assessor or the parent supports the standing infant by holding one or two hands. They encourage the infant to walk. Walking attempts may start with support of two hands, but gradually support of one hand is withdrawn. The assessor observes the motor behaviour of the infant.

RECORDING

Typical performance means that the infant takes at least four forward steps while being held by one hand (Fig. 5.73 and Video 5.108).

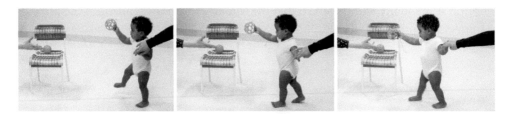

Figure 5.73 Walks when one hand held (Item 112)

Item 113   Squats With Support

POSITION

This item is assessed during standing (St).

PROCEDURE

The assessor or the parent puts an attractive object on a stool, a chair, or other relatively low piece of furniture. They encourage the infant to get the object. If the infant has pulled themselves into standing position, the assessor or parent puts an attractive object on the floor. They encourage the infant to get it. The assessor observes the motor behaviour of the infant.

RECORDING

Typical performance means that the infant squats while holding on to the furniture. The infant does not 'crash down' (Fig. 5.74 and Video 5.109).

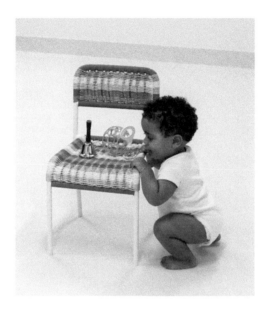

Figure 5.74 Squats with support (Item 113)

## CHAPTER 6

The Socio-Emotional Scale

INTRODUCTION

The Standardized Infant NeuroDevelopmental Assessment (SINDA) socio-emotional scale evaluates, with the help of six items, four types of behaviours: interaction, emotionality, self-regulation, and reactivity. These behaviours constitute the core set of the infant's temperament, i.e. the infant's set of reactivity and regulatory predispositions and the infant's characteristics that evolve in response to the environment, including complex social interactions (Jones and Sloan 2018). The evaluation of the items of the socio-emotional scale is based on the infant's behaviour during the assessment of the other two SINDA scales. Emotionality, self-regulation, and reactivity may be evaluated on the basis of the neurological scale only, but for the evaluation of interaction the items of the developmental scale are required.

General Remarks and Outcome Parameters

The assessment of the *interaction* between infant and adult (parent or assessor) is based on the age-specific cognitive and communication items of the developmental scale that are indicated by a red dot ●.

The items emotionality, self-regulation, and reactivity in response to change of position, and reactivity to visual stimuli and acoustic stimuli are scored at the end of the developmental assessment. These items are independent of the infant's age. Scoring of the emotionality, self-regulation, and reactivity items is based on the clinical impression of the infant's behaviour during the assessment and consists of a classification as typical (happy face icon: ☺) or atypical (sad face icon: ☹). The three reactivity items are used to generate a single reactivity classification, which is atypical when at least two of the three reactivity items have been scored as atypical.

SINDA's socio-emotional scale therefore results in a dichotomous score (typical vs atypical) on four types of specific behaviour: interaction, emotionality, self-regulation, and reactivity. The socio-emotional scale does not result in a total score. The interpretation of the socio-emotional items is discussed in Chapter 7.

DESCRIPTION OF THE ITEMS OF THE SOCIO-EMOTIONAL SCALE

Interaction

The infant's ability to interact with an adult refers to the infant's ability to experience, share, express, and regulate their affective state during interaction with the adult (Puura et al. 2019).

PROCEDURE

The assessment of the interaction between infant and adult (parent or assessor) is based on the age-specific cognitive and communication items of the developmental scale that are indicated by a red dot ● (see Figs 5.1 and 5.2).

SCORING

The proportion of the total number of age-specific 'red dot' items that the infant scored as 'pass' is calculated. For instance, at the age of 3 months three 'red dot' items are evaluated. If a 3-month-old infant has passed two of the three items, the infant's proportion of 'passed' items is 67%.

If the infant scores 'pass' on at least half ($\geq$50%) of the age-specific 'red dot' items, interaction is classified as typical (happy face icon: ☺), otherwise interaction is classified as atypical (sad face icon: ☹).

Emotionality

The infant's emotionality refers to the infant's ability to manage their arousal states (1) for affective biological and social adaptations, and (2) to achieve individual goals (Kopp and Neufeld 2003). The emotionality item evaluates the infant's mood during the assessment and is especially based on the infant's facial expressions and vocalizations.

PROCEDURE

The assessment of emotionality is based on the clinical impression during the entire assessment. Its final classification is determined at the end of the assessment.

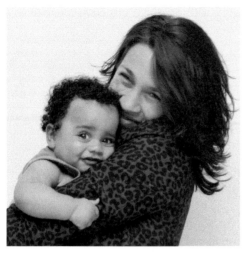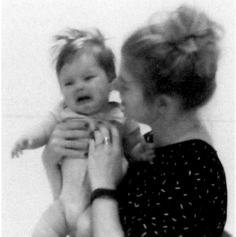

Figure 6.1 Typical (left) and atypical (right) emotionality

SCORING

Typical ☺   Smiles sometimes spontaneously and reactive to being talked to in a friendly way; reactive to being shown attractive objects; vocalizes with a positive expression; is in a happy mood most of the time; and is mostly relaxed (Fig. 6.1 and Video 6.1).

Atypical ☹   Shows predominantly a neutral or negative (frightened, irritated, sad) facial expression, even when being talked to in a friendly way or being presented with an attractive object; vocalizes with a negative expression (frightened, irritated, sad); and seems to be stressed most of the time (Fig. 6.1 and Video 6.1).

Self-Regulation

Self-regulation is the capacity to maintain attention, motor activity, and emotional state at a medium level in order to be able to explore, learn, and interact with the environment (Beeghly et al. 2016).

Self-regulation may occur unnoticed, i.e. without perceptible signs. When self-regulation is more challenging for the infant, clinical signs may occur. Facial expression may change into neutral or negative, and the infant may yawn. Vocalizations may change into fussing, crying, or pausing. Motor activity may change into increased sucking, pedalling, squirming, self-touching, intensive hand–hand contact, hand–mouth contact, or rocking. Behaviour may change, for instance, by avoiding or stopping contact, play, or communication, by moving eyes, head, or body away from the task or person, or by throwing objects away. Behavioural change may also include expression of the need for increased contact with parents, requesting soothing objects, such as a pacifier, or something to eat.

PROCEDURE

The assessment of self-regulation is based on the clinical impression during the entire assessment. Its final classification is determined at the end of the assessment.

SCORING

Typical ☺   Self-regulation allows for completion of the assessment; a temporary loss of the medium level of attention, motor activity, and emotional state may occur (Video 6.2).

Atypical ☹   Self-regulation does not allow for completion of the assessment or test completion requires intensive and long-lasting co-regulation of the investigator and parent. Co-regulation dominates the assessment (Video 6.2).

Reactivity

The compound item reactivity assesses the reactivity to visual, acoustic, and positional stimuli. Reactivity refers to the degree of inhibition of responses to environmental stimuli. Infants may be very inhibited, implying that they are hardly aroused by environmental stimuli, whereas other infants may be very uninhibited. The latter infants are easily aroused and respond to stimuli with high levels of motor activity, crying, smiling, or autonomic responses (Kagan 2013). The reactivity items evaluate the global impression of the latency and the intensity of the infant's responses to stimuli.

PROCEDURE

The assessment of reactivity is based on the clinical impression of reactivity to visual, acoustic, and positional stimuli during the entire assessment. The final classification of the reactivity items is determined at the end of the assessment. The three types of reactivity are first scored separately, according to the following criteria.

SCORING

Typical ☺   Reacts to moderate stimuli with typical latency (about 1 second) with pausing, moving happily, eye opening, listening, increasing alertness, vocalizing, increasing motor activity, moving eyes or head in the direction of the stimulus, smiling (Video 6.3).

Atypical ☹   Shows at least one of the following reactions (Video 6.3):
- reacts even to a very low stimulus intensity
- reacts only to a very high stimulus intensity
- reactions consistently delayed (with a latency of more than 2 seconds)

- does not react at all (note: deafness, severe hearing impairment, blindness, or severe visual impairment should be excluded)
- reacts too fast (within a split second)
- reacts as frightened or with irritation, crying, jittering, or opisthotonos.

The compound reactivity is determined on the basis of the scores of the three reactivity items. Reactivity is atypical when at least two of the three reactivity items have been scored as atypical.

## CHAPTER 7

Significance of SINDA Findings

THE AIMS OF SINDA

Standardized Infant NeuroDevelopmental Assessment (SINDA) has been designed as a screening instrument for infants aged 6 weeks to 12 months to detect infants who are at high risk of a neurological and/or developmental disorder. The instrument can be used by any health professional involved in the early detection of developmental disorders, for instance paediatricians, developmental paediatricians, child neurologists, paediatric physiotherapists, and occupational and speech therapists.

SINDA provides health professionals with information on the infant's current neurodevelopmental status in terms of the infant's neurological condition, the presence or absence of a developmental delay, and the infant's socio-emotional characteristics. This information assists parent counselling and the determination of the infant's risk of neurodevelopmental disorders, including cerebral palsy, intellectual disability, and emotional and behavioural disorders.

The current chapter discusses the significance of SINDA's findings. It starts with the neurological scale. Then the developmental scale and the socio-emotional scale are discussed. The discussion of the scales includes a short description of the findings in the Dutch norm study, i.e. the study on 1100 infants aged 6 weeks to 12 months representative of the Dutch population in terms of perinatal and social background characteristics, including maternal education and ethnicity (Straathof et al. 2020; Wu et al. 2020; see Chapter 3). Concluding remarks complete the chapter.

SINDA'S NEUROLOGICAL SCALE

SINDA's neurological scale contains items of the five major infant neurological domains: spontaneous movements, cranial nerves, motor reactions to postural stimulation, muscle tone, and reflexes and reactions. SINDA's neurological scale pays substantially more attention to the quality of the infant's spontaneous movements than other infant neurological assessments, such as the Hammersmith Infant Neurological Examination (HINE; Romeo et al. 2016) and the Amiel-Tison Neurological Assessment (Amiel-Tison and Grenier 1986; for an overview see Majnemer et al. 2021). The decision to include a relatively large proportion (7 of the 28 items; 25%) of items on the quality of spontaneous movements was based on the accumulating evidence that the quality of spontaneous movements is a major marker of the infant's brain integrity and greatly assists the prediction of developmental outcome (Prechtl 1990; Chapter 3). Due to its inclusion of the relatively high proportion of spontaneous movements, SINDA's neurological scale not only predicts high risk of cerebral palsy, but also of intellectual disability (Hadders-Algra et al. 2019).

Table 7.1 provides an overview of the prevalence of atypical performance on the 28 items of SINDA's neurological scale in the Dutch normative population. The prevalence of atypical performance with some items (pupillary reaction, tendon reflexes, foot sole sensibility, and foot sole response) is low (≤2%). For other items the prevalence of atypical performance is relatively high (25–35%). The latter is true for vertical suspension, feet touching the ground, and muscle tone of arms, legs, and feet. The findings indicate that many infants have an atypical muscle tone in one part of the body. This corresponds to the notion that atypical muscle tone only has clinical significance when it occurs in multiple parts of the body (Harris 2008; Straathof et al. 2021). Expressed more generally, a single sign of atypical neurological performance usually has no clinical relevance.[1] Signs of atypical neurological performance generally only have clinical significance when they co-occur with other signs of atypical neurological performance and form a neurologically meaningful pattern. Examples of such patterns are a consistent asymmetry in spontaneous movements, muscle tone, and reflexes and reactions, and the pattern consisting of the combination of stereotyped movements in many parts of the body, atypical motor reactions to postural stimulation, atypical muscle tone, and atypical reflexes. The nervous system's characteristic to express clinically relevant impairment in an accumulation of atypical neurological signs explains why only a significant reduction of SINDA's neurological score (>7 of its 28 points; the atypical score of ≤21) is associated with a highly increased risk of neurological and/or developmental disorders (Hadders-Algra et al. 2019; Hadders-Algra 2020).

Our studies demonstrated that SINDA's neurological scale has very good predictive properties in the setting of an outpatient clinic of at-risk infants (Hadders-Algra et al.

---

[1] We wrote 'usually has no clinical relevance' as exceptions to this rule may occur. A case in point is the single sign of an asymmetric pupillary reaction, which may be the first sign of severe intracranial pathology such as a brain tumour.

Table 7.1 Prevalence of atypical neurological items in Dutch population norms

SINDA Neurological Scale
prevalence of atypical scores in the Dutch population norms
(*n*=1100 infants, 2–12 months)

Item number	Item	Typical (1)	Atypical (0)	Prevalence of atypical score *n* (%)	
A1 Spontaneous movements (local)					
1	Head & neck & trunk	varied & symmetric	stereotyped posture, opisthotonus, asymmetric	58	(5.3%)
2	Arms	varied & symmetric	stereotyped posture, asymmetric	165	(15.0%)
3	Hands	varied & symmetric	stereotyped posture, asymmetric	121	(11.0%)
4	Legs	varied & symmetric	stereotyped posture, asymmetric	86	(7.8%)
5	Feet	varied & symmetric	stereotyped posture, asymmetric	52	(4.7%)
6	ATNR	absent, occasionally present	frequently, continuously present, asymmetric	32	(2.9%)
A2 Spontaneous movements (general)					
7	Quality	varied & symmetric & fluent & isolated movements of fingers & toes	stereotyped, jerky, jittery, startles, tremulous, sluggish, stiff, no isolated movements of fingers, toes, asymmetric	52	(4.7%)
8	Quantity	moderate & changing over time	predominantly hypokinetic, predominantly hyperkinetic	38	(3.5%)
B Cranial nerves					
9	Facial appearance	varied & symmetric	expressionless, asymmetric	38	(3.5%)
10	Oral motor behaviour	mouth mostly closed & tongue within the mouth & no obvious drooling	mouth mostly open, stereotyped tongue protrusion, fasciculations, obvious drooling	214	(19.5%)
11	Glabella reflex	moderate threshold & moderate intensity & symmetric	low, high threshold, low, high intensity, asymmetric	19	(1.7%)
12	Eye position & eye movements	fixates & parallel position & conjugated movements	no fixation, predominant strabism, unconjugated movements, restricted motility, sunset, nystagmus	35	(3.2%)
13	Optical blink reflex	blinks & symmetric	absent, doubtful, delayed, asymmetric	190	(17.3%)
14	Pupillary reaction	direct & indirect: prompt & symmetric	absent, slow, tonic, asymmetric	16	(1.5%)
15	Acoustic reaction to clapping	blinks, facial reaction	absent, doubtful	109	(9.9%)
C Motor reactions to postural stimulation					
16	Pull-to-sit	activation of neck & shoulder & arm muscles & symmetric arm activity & adequate flexion hips	head lag, active retroflexion, no or minimal muscle activation, asymmetric, inadequate hipflexion	196	(17.8%)
17	Head in prone	lifts head as selective action	does not lift head, stereotyped hyperextension	50	(4.5%)
18	Prone suspension	head in line, above trunk level	head, trunk floppy, stereotyped, opisthotonus	65	(5.9%)
19	Vertical suspension	head upright & appropriate axillary resistance & legs varied & symmetric	poor head control, slipping through, stereotyped leg movements, asymmetric	345	(31.4%)
20	Feet touching the ground	varied feet postures & movements & symmetric	stereotyped feet postures, asymmetric	293	(26.6%)
D Muscle tone					
21	Tone of neck & trunk	moderate resistance against passive movements	consistent hypotonia, consistent hypertonia, sudden changes in muscle tone	59	(5.4%)
22	Resistance against passive movements, arm traction	symmetric & moderate resistance against passive movements & slight elbow flexion	consistent hypotonia, consistent hypertonia, sudden changes in muscle tone, asymmetric	312	(28.4%)
23	Resistance against passive movements, leg traction	symmetric & moderate resistance against passive movements & slight knee flexion	consistent hypotonia, consistent hypertonia, sudden changes in muscle tone, asymmetric	353	(32.1%)
24	Feet: resistance against passive movements	symmetric & moderate resistance against passive movements	consistent hypotonia, consistent hypertonia, sudden changes in muscle tone, ankle clonus, positive catch phenomenon, asymmetric	295	(26.8%)
E Reflexes and reactions					
25	Upper extremities: biceps reflex	symmetric positive response	areflexia, asymmetric	5	(0.5%)
26	Lower extremities: knee jerk & ankle clone	symmetric positive response	areflexia, tonic response, clonic, asymmetric	20	(1.8%)
27	Foot sole sensibility	withdrawal of legs & varied toe movement & symmetric	no reaction, stereotyped toe movements, asymmetric	22	(2.0%)
28	Foot sole response	varied dorsiflexion 1st toe & toe spreading & symmetric	stereotyped, tonic dorsi- or plantar flexion, no or weak response, asymmetric	20	(1.8%)

ATNR, asymmetrical tonic neck response.

2019; Hadders-Algra 2020). The atypical neurological score (≤21) predicted cerebral palsy with a sensitivity of 91% to 100% and a specificity of 81% to 85%; it predicted cerebral palsy and/or intellectual disability with a sensitivity of 83% to 89% and a specificity of 94% to 96% (Table 3.3). The properties of SINDA's neurological scale to predict cerebral palsy and intellectual disability are comparable to those of the HINE (Romeo et al. 2021). Yet, it should be noted that HINE is more difficult to apply as its criteria for atypical item performance are age-dependent and its criteria for an atypical neurological score are only available for a limited number of infant ages (Hadders-Algra 2021a).

However, predictive properties of neurodevelopmental instruments in groups of at-risk infants always outperform the predictive properties of the same instruments in the general population. Usually, the latter is not studied, as it requires relatively large groups of infants representative of the general population. To the best of our knowledge only the prediction of atypical general movements in 3-month-old infants has been studied both in high-risk groups and in the general population (Bouwstra et al. 2010; Bosanquet et al. 2013; De Bock et al. 2017). Bouwstra et al.'s study (2010) demonstrated that the predictive power of general movement assessment in the general population was good but less robust than that in high-risk groups.

We would like to emphasize that the notion of 'at risk' does not imply certainty. Rather, it induces uncertainty. Due to the high rate of developmental changes in the nervous system during infancy, the neurological condition may change. It may improve, and it may deteriorate with increasing age, i.e. the infant may grow out of or into a neurological impairment (see Chapter 2; Fig. 2.1). This uncertainty has major implications for parental counselling and parental support during early intervention. The uncertainty and the absence of a diagnosis do, however, not preclude the need for early intervention (Hadders-Algra 2021b). On the contrary, the presence of an atypical neurological score is an indication for early intervention.

The presence of an atypical neurological score (≤21) means that the infant currently has a significant neurological impairment. The impairment invokes the need of three actions:

- The cause of the impairment needs to be assessed. The infant's prenatal, perinatal, neonatal, developmental, and family history may provide clues. In addition, and depending on the infant's history and clinical picture, other assessments are performed, such as neuroimaging (cranial ultrasound or magnetic resonance imaging), electro-encephalography (or other neurophysiological assessments), or a metabolic screen.

- The family is informed and counselled about the infant's current status, including the difficult notion of 'at risk'. The latter notion implies that early intervention is recommended.

- The implementation of early intervention. Current early intervention programmes are family centred. They focus on (1) support of parents, including support to deal with the uncertainty of the infant's 'at-risk' status, and (2) stimulation of infant activities. The infant activities are not restricted to the mobility domain but also address learning and communication (Hadders-Algra 2021b).

Table 7.2 Prevalence of typical developmental items in infants aged 2 to 6 months in the Dutch normative population

SINDA developmental scale
prevalence of typical scores in the Dutch normative population
(2–6 months, 100 infants per month)

#	1 M 15 - **2 M** - 2 M 14	*n*	#	2 M 15 - **3 M** - 3 M 14	*n*	#	3 M 15 - **4 M** - 4 M 14	*n*	#	4 M 15 - **5 M** - 5 M 14	*n*	#	5 M 15 - **6 M** - 6 M 14	*n*
1	Smiles in response to smile of parent or assessor	87	16	Looks alternately from parents to assessor	57	16	Looks alternately from parents to assessor	64	27	Interested in environment and objects in room	100	49	Inspects facial expression of assessor with sustained attention	99
2	Initiates contact with assessor, explores face and facial expression	89	4	Produces ≥2 different sounds (e.g. gaah, ooh)	81	27	Interested in environment and objects in room	99	28	Looks alternately from object to person	99	50	Uses facial expressions to communicate	97
3	Reacts to cooing-like expressions of parent or assessor	79	5	Produces sounds as dialogue when being talked to	69	28	Looks alternately from object to person	73	31	Produces sounds to express emotions, laughs loudly	50	39	Produces ≥3 consonant–vowel combinations	34
4	Produces ≥2 different sounds (e.g. gaah, ooh)	75	17	Produces sounds with expression: expresses emotions	66	29	Produces ≥3 different sounds	60	39	Localizes ≥3 consonant–vowel combinations	12	51	Produces sounds to attract attention to themself	84
5	Produces sounds as dialogue when being talked to	71	18	Blinks in response to optical approach of hand	90	30	Produces ≥1 labial consonant and one consonant–vowel combination	17	40	Localizes voices & directs visual attention to voice	94	52	Produces strings of syllables with speech melody	27
6	Reacts to sound	93	19	Turns eyes to sound-producing object	69	31	Produces sounds to express emotions, laughs loudly	43	32	Visually searches to find object that disappeared	78	53	Turns eyes or head to soft sound, e.g. rustling of paper	96
7	Briefly fixates object at 30cm distance	91	20	Turns visual attention slowly from one 'sound object' to another	38	20	Turns visual attention slowly from one 'sound object' to another	61	41	Looks ≥3 sec in direction of hidden object	34	41	Looks ≥3 sec in direction of hidden object	42
8	Follows object with eyes or head horizontally	89	21	Follows object with eyes or head, horizontally and vertically	90	32	Visually searches to find object that disappeared	62	42	Visually explores an object held in their hand	68	54	Visually observes falling and 'crashing' object	77
9	Follows object with eyes or head vertically	91	11	Inspects own hand	28	12	Moves arm in direction of attractive object	88	43	Reaches across midline	74	55	Explores object with interest for details	52
10	Moves hand to mouth	57	22	Moves arm at appearance of object within visual field	93	33	Grasps object presented within visual fields with hand	73	44	Transfers object from one hand to the other	61	44	Transfers object from one hand to the other	86
11	Inspects own hand	10	12	Moves arm in direction of attractive object	63	34	Brings object to mouth, & explores with mouth and hand	51	45	Holds one object & reaches and touches a second object	78	45	Holds one object & reaches and touches a second object	97
12	Moves arm in direction of attractive object	26	23	Hands in midline & touching of hands	52	35	Explores object with both hands	52	46	Plays with string	52	56	Briefly holds two grasped objects	95
13	Balances head for ≥3 sec in supported sitting	87	24	Balances head for ≥5 sec in supported sitting	85	36	Balances head for ≥10 sec in supported sitting, some wobbling allowed	92	37	Hand touches knee	68	57	Plays with foot (hand–foot contact)	55
14	Lifts legs alternately on support surface & lifted bilaterally for ≥3 sec	87	25	Legs lifted from support surface with ≥3 sec foot-foot contact	59	37	Hand touches knee	49	47	Supported on two elbows & attempts to obtain object	50	58	Wriggling	86
15	Lifts head: chin off support surface for ≥3 sec	68	26	Lifts head >45° for ≥3 sec	60	38	Lifts head >45° with elbow support ≥5 sec	68	48	Stable head position in supported sitting	79	59	'Stands' on hands, unilaterally or bilaterally	57

Table 7.3 Prevalence of typical developmental items in infants aged 7 to 12 months in the Dutch normative population

SINDA developmental scale
prevalence of typical scores in the Dutch normative population
(7–12 months, 100 infants per month)

6 M 15 - 7 M - 7 M 14

#	Item	n
60	Observes with interest peek-a-boo play	88 ●
61	Shows referential gazing	90 ●
52	Strings of syllables with speech melody	40
62	Identifies desires with gestures or facial expressions	88 ●
63	Imitates consonant–vowel sequences	5
54	Visually observes falling and 'crashing' object	90 ●
64	Pays visual attention to scribbling	77
65	Produces sound by hitting with object	70
66	Grasps & holds two objects ≥3 sec	96
67	Intentionally pulls string to obtain object	65
68	Uses scissor grasp	13
69	Sits independantly for ≥3 sec	65
70	Turns from supine into prone	69
71	Reaches out for object in prone	98
72	Pivots	64

7 M 15 - 8 M - 8 M 14

#	Item	n
60	Observes with interest peek-a-boo play	95
73	Imitates e.g. clapping of hands or waving	44 ●
74	Responses to clear 'no'	52 ●
52	Strings of syllables with speech melody	71
62	Identifies desires with gestures or facial expressions	95
63	Imitates consonant– vowel sequences	17
75	Anticipatory gaze to object reappearance	50
76	Looks at pictures in book	77
77	Turns object to explore it visually	99
67	Intentionally pulls string to obtain object	87
78	Tries to pick object from cup	81
69	Sits independantly for ≥3 sec	93
79	Gets on all fours independently	38
80	Progression, e.g. abdominal crawling, rolling	53

8 M 15 - 9 M - 9 M 14

#	Item	n
73	Imitates e.g. clapping of hands or waving	54
74	Responses to clear 'no'	56 ●
81	Produces chains of three syllables (canonical babbling)	52
82	Responses to own name	50 ●
75	Anticipatory gaze to object reappearance	46
76	Looks at pictures in book	99
83	Intentionally rings bell	77
67	Intentionally pulls string to obtain object	96
84	Removes obstacle to get object	86
85	Explores details of object with fingertips	79
86	Puts object in cup	32
87	Sits independently for sustained periods of time	92
88	Sits independently and rotates trunk	63
89	Stands on knees while holding on to furniture	42
90	Progression on all fours, bunny hop, bottom shuffling	32

9 M 15 - 10 M - 10 M 14

#	Item	n
91	Imitates play of 'clap your hands' or other hand or finger play	24
92	Uses different expressions or gestures for known and unknown persons	85
82	Responds to own name	57 ●
93	Responds to question: 'Where is...?' (object, person)	30 ●
94	Produces ≥ 2 different chains of three syllables	51
83	Intentionally rings bell	87
95	Looks at pictures in book & turns pages	84
96	Engages in joint exploration (joint attention)	84 ●
85	Explores details of object with fingertips	84
86	Puts object in cup	50
97	Uses index finger to touch details of object	70
88	Sits independently and rotates trunk	75
90	Progression on all fours, bunny hop, bottom shuffling	60
98	Gets into sitting position independently	58
99	Pulls to stand	57

10 M 15 - 11 M - 11 M 14

#	Item	n
91	Imitates play of 'clap your hands' or other hand or finger play	48 ●
92	Responds to own name	72 ●
93	Responds to question: 'Where is...?' (object, person)	38 ●
94	≥2 different chains of three syllables	66
83	Intentionally rings bell	92
95	Looks at pictures in book & turns pages	91
96	Engages in joint exploration (joint attention)	95
100	Finds object covered by cup	84
97	Uses index finger to touch details of object	92
101	Holds two objects & grasps third object	49
102	Uses spoon to stir in cup or on plate (in imitation)	23
103	Pulls the right string to retrieve object	65
90	Progression on all fours, bunny hop, bottom shuffling	80
99	Pulls to stand	74
104	Cruises along furniture	64

11 M 15 - 12 M - 12 M 14

#	Item	n
93	Responds to question: 'Where is...?' (object, person)	47 ●
105	Shows semantic gestures when challenged	68 ●
106	Uses 'mama' or 'dada' or other meaningful word	36 ●
95	Looks at pictures in book & turns pages	99
96	Engages in joint exploration (joint attention)	87 ●
107	Finds object hidden under one of two cups	70
108	Points with index finger to persons or objects	58 ●
101	Holds two objects & grasps third object	45
102	Uses spoon to stir in cup or on plate (in imitation)	36
103	Pulls the right string to retrieve object	65
109	Uses pincer grasp	89
110	Throws small ball forward	67
111	Stands independently for ≥3 sec	35
112	Walks when one hand held	43
113	Squats with support	52

SINDA'S DEVELOPMENTAL SCALE

SINDA's developmental scale contains 15 items per testing month that are representative of the infant's performance in the domains of cognition, communication, and gross and fine motor skills. The Dutch normative study showed that the item set of each month contains items that are relatively easy and items that are relatively difficult (Tables 7.2 and 7.3). Some items belong to multiple month-specific item sets. In the item set of the youngest testing month the recurring items are relatively difficult, whereas they are relatively easy in the item set of the oldest testing month. Item 52 ('produces strings of syllables with speech melody') may serve as an example. It is assessed at 6, 7, and 8 months. The proportion of infants of the Dutch normative population achieving this ability increases from 27% at 6 months, to 40% at 7 months, and 71% at 8 months (Tables 7.2 and 7.3).

The developmental scale's primary aim is parent counselling. The scale provides information on the presence or absence of a global developmental delay or a domain specific limitation, i.e. a specific limitation in cognition, communication, and fine or gross motor abilities. If the assessment of the developmental scale indicates that the infant has an atypical score (≤ 7), assessment of the item sets of younger ages may provide information about the infant's current level of performance and therewith furnish an estimate of the infant's developmental delay. This information helps parents to understand their infant's performances and behaviour during daily life. The developmental information is also essential background information in early intervention (Hadders-Algra 2021b).

The atypical developmental score (≤ 7) also assists prediction. It primarily assists the prediction of intellectual disability. The atypical developmental score predicted the presence of intellectual disability at the age of at least 2 years with a sensitivity of 77% and a specificity of 92%. The developmental score has also been validated for use in infants with trisomy 21. In these infants the developmental score may assist with the counselling of parents of infants as the score provides information about the infant's abilities. Finally, the combination of an atypical score on the neurological and the developmental scale further improves the already highly predictive properties of SINDA's neurological scale for atypical developmental outcome. The presence of atypical scores on both scales is virtually always associated with atypical developmental outcome (Hadders-Algra et al. 2020).

SINDA'S SOCIO-EMOTIONAL SCALE

SINDA's socio-emotional scale furnishes information on four aspects of infant behaviour: interaction, emotionality, self-regulation, and reactivity to various stimuli. The Dutch normative study indicated that the prevalence of atypical socio-emotional behaviour is: interaction 17%, emotionality 14%, self-regulation 10%, and reactivity 1%.

The primary aim of the socio-emotional scale is parent counselling. Parent counselling serves to support parents with how to interact with their infant. This not only assists parents in being able to interact sensitively with their infant during daily care-giving activities but also reduces the chance of the infant being diagnosed with an emotional and behavioural disorder at a later age (Thomas et al. 2017). Infants thrive through ongoing experiences with caregivers that adapt their behaviour in an empathic, consistent, and contingently responsive way. The sensitive interactions help the infant to understand and structure their world (Clark et al. 2020).

Two of SINDA's socio-emotional behaviours have predictive value. Atypical emotionality and atypical self-regulation predicted the presence of an emotional or behavioural disorder at the age of at least 2 years with a high specificity (85% and 98%, respectively), but a relatively low sensitivity (32% and 40%, respectively; Hadders-Algra et al. 2020). The relatively low sensitivity illustrates the multifactorial origin of emotional and behavioural disorders (Kostyrka-Allchorne et al. 2020). Nonetheless, the findings also imply that infants with atypical emotionality or atypical self-regulation have a substantial risk of being diagnosed with an emotional or behavioural disorder later in life. On the other hand, typical emotionality and typical self-regulation do not preclude the development of an emotional or behavioural disorder. Yet, typical emotionality and typical self-regulation form important sources of resilience for the infant to cope with daily life experiences (Beeghly et al. 2016; Clark et al. 2020).

CONCLUDING REMARKS

SINDA is a screening instrument that can be reliably and relatively easily and quickly applied in infants aged 6 weeks to 12 months. SINDA's ease is based on (1) the age-independent set of 28 neurological and six socio-emotional items and the age-specific set of 15 developmental items, and (2) the age-independent cut-off criteria for atypical performance. The latter is an important difference with the HINE, which has age-dependent cut-offs that have only been established for the ages of 3, 6, 9, and 12 months and that vary between publications (Romeo et al. 2016).

SINDA primarily provides health professionals with information on the infant's current neurodevelopmental and socio-emotional status. This information is quintessential for parent counselling. Second, SINDA furnishes information on the infant's risk of neurodevelopmental disorders, such as cerebral palsy, intellectual disability, and emotional or behavioural disorders. It is important to realize that SINDA does not result in a specific neurodevelopmental diagnosis. Rather, the findings of SINDA may invoke the need of further diagnostics, including longitudinal monitoring of the infant's development. The latter is inherent to the characteristics of the young developing brain. The infant's brain plasticity may induce a transient or permanent improvement of the infant's function, but it may also result in an impairment that becomes increasingly clear with increasing age (Chapter 2; Reuner and Pietz 2006; Heineman and Hadders-Algra 2008).

References

Alam S, Lux AL (2012) Epilepsies in infancy. *Arch Dis Child* **97**: 985–992.

Amiel-Tison C, Grenier A (1986) *Neurological Assessment During the First Year of Life*. Oxford: Oxford University Press.

Bayley N (1993) *Manual of the Bayley Scales of Infant Development*, 2nd edn. San Antonio: The Psychological Corporation.

Bayley N (2006) *Manual of the Bayley Scales of Infant and Toddler Development*, 3rd edn. San Antonio: The Psychological Corporation.

Beeghly M, Perry BD, Tronick E (2016) Self-regulatory processes in early development. In: Maltzman S (ed.) *The Oxford Handbook of Treatment Processes and Outcomes in Psychology: a Multidisciplinary, Biopsychosocial Approach*. Oxford: Oxford Handbooks Online, doi: 10.1093/oxfordhb/9780199739134.013.3.

Berger R, Michaelis R (2009) Neurologische Basisuntersuchung für das Alter von 0–2 Jahren. Die Items. *Monatsschr Kinderheilkunde* **157**: 1103–1112.

Bohlin G, Hagekull B (2009) Socio-emotional development: from infancy to young adulthood. *Scand J Psychol* **50**: 592–601.

Bosanquet M, Copeland L, Ware R et al. (2013) A systematic review of tests to predict cerebral palsy in young children. *Dev Med Child Neurol* **55**: 418–426.

Bouwstra H, Dijck-Stigter GR, Grooten HMJ et al. (2010) Predictive value of definitely abnormal GMs at three months in the general population. *Dev Med Child Neurol* **52**: 456–461.

Bruijn SM, Massaad F, Maclellan MJ et al. (2013) Are effects of the symmetric and asymmetric tonic neck reflexes still visible in healthy adults? *Neurosci Lett* **556**: 89–92.

Chawanpaiboon S, Vogel JP, Moller AB et al. (2019) Global, regional, and national estimates of levels of preterm birth in 2014: a systematic review and modelling analysis. *Lancet Glob Health* **7**: e37–e46.

Cignetti F, Zedka M, Vaugoyeau M et al. (2013) Independent walking as a major skill for the development of anticipatory postural control: evidence from adjustments to predictable perturbations. *PLoS One* **8**: e56313.

Clark R, Tluczek A, Moore EC et al. (2020) Theoretical and empirical foundations for early relationship assessment in evaluating infant and toddler mental health. In: DelCarmen R, Carter AS (eds) *The Oxford Handbook of Infant, Toddler, and Preschool Mental Health Assessment*, 2nd ed. Oxford: Oxford Handbooks Online, doi: 10.1093/oxfordhb/9780199837182.013.2.

Dan B, Mayston M, Paneth N et al. (2014) *Cerebral Palsy: Science and Clinical Practice*. London: Mac Keith Press.

Deciphering Developmental Disorders Study (2015) Large-scale discovery of novel genetic causes of developmental disorders. *Nature* **519**: 223–228.

De Bock F, Will H, Behrenbeck U et al. (2017) Predictive value of General Movement Assessment for preterm infants' development at 2 years – implementation in clinical routine in a non-academic setting. *Res Dev Disabilities* **62**: 69–80.

De Graaf-Peters VB, Hadders-Algra M (2006) Ontogeny of the human central nervous system: What is happening when? *Early Hum Dev* **82**: 257–266.

Eyre JA (2007) Corticospinal tract development and its plasticity after perinatal injury. *Neurosci Biobehav Rev* **31**: 1136–1149.

Granild-Jensen JB, Rackauskaite G, Flachs EM et al. (2015) Predictors for early diagnosis of cerebral palsy from national registry data. *Dev Med Child Neurol* **57**: 931–935.

Green E, Stroud L, Bloomfield S et al. (2015) *Griffiths Scales of Child Development*, 3rd edn. Amsterdam: Hogrefe.

Haataja L, Mercuri E, Regev R et al. (1999) Optimality score for the neurologic examination of the infant at 12 and 18 months of age. *J Pediatr* **135**: 153–161.

Hadders-Algra M (2002) Two distinct forms of minor neurological dysfunction: perspectives emerging from a review of data of the Groningen Perinatal Project. *Dev Med Child Neurol* **44**: 561–571.

Hadders-Algra M (2004) General movements: a window for early identification of children at high risk of developmental disorders. *J Pediatr* **145**: S12–S18.

Hadders-Algra M (2018a) Early human brain development: starring the subplate. *Neurosci Biobehav Rev* **92**: 276–290.

Hadders-Algra M (2018b) Early human motor development: from variation to the ability to vary and adapt. *Neurosci Biobehav Rev* **90**: 411–427.

Hadders-Algra M (2018c) Neural substrate and clinical significance of general movements: an update. *Dev Med Child Neurol* **60**: 39–46.

Hadders-Algra M (2021a) Early diagnostics and early intervention in neurodevelopmental disorders – age-dependent challenges and opportunities. *J Clin Med* **10**: 861.

Hadders-Algra M (2021b) Early intervention in the first two years post-termt. In: Hadders-Algra M (ed.) *Early Detection and Early Intervention in Developmental Motor Disorders – From Neuroscience to Participation*. London: Mac Keith Press, pp. 198–227.

Hadders-Algra M, Heineman KR, Bos AF et al. (2010) The assessment of minor neurological dysfunction using the Touwen Infant Neurological Examination: strengths and limitations. *Dev Med Child Neurol* **52**: 87–92.

Hadders-Algra M, Boxum AG, Hielkema T et al. (2017) Effect of early intervention in infants at very high risk of cerebral palsy – a systematic review. *Dev Med Child Neurol* **59**: 246–258.

Hadders-Algra M, Tacke U, Pietz J et al. (2019) Reliability and predictive validity of the Standardized Infant NeuroDevelopmental Assessment neurological scale. *Dev Med Child Neurol* **61**: 654–660.

Hadders-Algra M, Tacke U, Pietz J et al. (2020) Standardized Infant NeuroDevelopmental Assessment developmental and socio-emotional scales: reliability and predictive value in an at risk population. *Dev Med Child Neurol* **62**: 845–853.

Hamer EG, Vermeulen RJ, Dijkstra LJ et al. (2016) Slow pupillary light responses in infants at high risk of cerebral palsy were associated with periventricular leukomalacia and neurological outcome. *Acta Paediatr* **105**: 1493–1501.

Hamer E, La Bastide-Van Gemert S, Boxum A et al. (2018) The tonic response to the infant knee jerk as an early sign of cerebral palsy. *Early Hum Dev* **119**: 38–44.

Harris SR (2008) Congenital hypotonia: clinical and developmental assessment. *Dev Med Child Neurol* **50**: 889–892.

Haynes RL, Borenstein NS, DesilvaTM et al. (2005) Axonal development in the cerebral white matter of the human fetus and infant. *J Comp Neurol* **484**: 156–167.

Heineman KR, Hadders-Algra M (2008) Evaluation of neuromotor function in infancy – a systematic review of available methods. *J Dev Behav Pediatr* **29**: 315–323.

Heineman KR, Bos AF, Hadders-Algra M (2011) Infant motor profile and cerebral palsy: promising associations. *Dev Med Child Neurol* **53**(4): 40–45.

Herlenius E, Lagercrantz H (2010) Neurotransmitters and neuromodulators. In: Lagercrantz H, Hanson MA, Ment LR et al. (eds) *The Newborn Brain. Neuroscience and Clinical Applications*, 2nd edn. Cambridge: Cambridge University Press, pp. 99–117.

Jones NA, Sloan A (2018) Neurohormones and temperament interact during infant development. *Philos Trans R Soc Lond B Biol Sci* **373**: 20170159.

Kagan J (2013) Temperamental contributions to inhibited and uninhibited profiles. In: Zelazo PD (ed.) *The Oxford Handbook of Developmental Psychology, Vol. 2: Self and Other*. Oxford: Oxford Handbooks Online, doi: 10.1093/oxfordhb/9780199958474.013.0007.

Kopp CB, Neufeld SJ (2003) Emotional development during infancy. In: Davidson RJ, Scherer KR, Goldsmith HH (eds) *Handbook of Affective Sciences*. Oxford: Oxford University Press, pp. 347–374.

Kostović I, Judas M (2010) The development of the subplate and thalamocortical connections in the human foetal brain. *Acta Paediatr* **99**: 1119–1127.

Kostović I, Jovanov-Milošević N, Radoš M et al. (2014a) Perinatal and early postnatal reorganization of the subplate and related cellular components in the human cerebral wall as revealed by histological and MRI approaches. *Brain Struct Funct* **219**: 231–253.

Kostović I, Kostović-Srzentić M, Benjak V et al. (2014b) Developmental dynamics of radial vulnerability in the cerebral compartments in preterm infants and neonates. *Front Neurol* **5**: 139.

Kostović I, Sedmak G, Vukšić M et al. (2015) The relevance of human fetal subplate zone for developmental neuropathology of neuronal migration disorders and cortical dysplasia CNS. *Neurosci Ther* **21**: 74–82.

Kostyrka-Allchorne K, Wass SV, Sonuga-Barke EJS (2020) Research review: do parent ratings of infant negative emotionality and self-regulation predict psychopathology in childhood and adolescence? A systematic review and meta-analysis of prospective longitudinal studies. *J Child Psychol Psychiatry* **61**: 401–416.

Lossi L, Merighi A (2003) In vivo cellular and molecular mechanisms of neuronal apoptosis in the mammalian CNS. *Prog Neurobiol* **69**: 287–312.

Magnus R, de Kleijn A (1912) Die Abhängigkeit des Tonus der Extremitätenmusklen von der Kopfstellung. *Pflüger's Arch* **145**: 455–548.

Majnemer A, Snider L, Hadders-Algra M (2021) Assessment of infants and toddlers. In: Hadders-Algra M (ed.) *Early Detection and Early Intervention in Developmental Motor Disorders – From Neuroscience to Participation in Daily Life*. London: Mac Keith Press, pp. 144–170.

Michaelis R, Berger R (2007) Neurologische Basisuntersuchung für das Alter von 0–2 Jahren. Ein Konsensusvorschlag. *Monatsschr Kinderheilkunde* **155**: 506–513.

Michaelis R, Asenbauer C, Buchwald-Saal M et al. (1993) Transitory neurological findings in a population of at risk infants. *Early Hum Dev* **34**: 143–153.

Miller SL, Huppi PS, Mallard C (2016) The consequences of fetal growth restriction on brain structure and neurodevelopmental outcome. *J Physiol* **594**: 807–823.

Mullen EM (1995) *Mullen Scales of Early Learning*. Circle Pines, MN: American Guidance Service.

Mwaniki MK, Atieno M, Lawn JE et al. (2012) Long-term neurodevelopmental outcomes after intrauterine and neonatal insults: a systematic review. *Lancet* **379**: 445–452.

Nuysink J, Eijsermans MJ, van Haastert IC et al. (2013) Clinical course of asymmetric motor performance and deformational plagiocephaly in very preterm infants. *J Pediatr* **163**: 658–665.

Ozonoff S, Iosif AM, Baguio F et al. (2010) A prospective study of the emergence of early behavioral signs of autism. *J Am Acad Child Adolesc Psychiatry* **49**: 256–266.

Peiper A (1963) *Cerebral Function in Infancy and Childhood*, 3rd edn. New York: Consultants Bureau.

Petanjek Z, Judaš M, Šimic G et al. (2011) Extraordinary neoteny of synaptic spines in the human prefrontal cortex. *Proc Natl Acad Sci USA* **108**: 13281–13286.

Prechlt HFR (1977) *The Neurological Examination of the Full Term Newborn*, 2nd edn. London: Heinemann Medical Books.

Prechtl HFR (1990) Qualitative changes of spontaneous movements in fetus and preterm infant are a marker of neurological dysfunction. *Early Hum Dev* **23**: 151–158.

Puura K, Leppänen J, Salmelin R et al. (2019) Maternal and infant characteristics connected to shared pleasure in dyadic interaction. *Infant Ment Health J* **40**: 459–478.

Reuner G, Pietz J (2006) Entwicklungsdiagnostik im Säuglings- und Kleinkindalter. *Monatsschr Kinderheilkd* **154**: 305–313.

Romeo DM, Ricci D, Brogna C et al. (2016) Use of the Hammersmith Infant Neurological Examination in infant with cerebral palsy: a critical review of the literature. *Dev Med Child Neurol* **58**: 240–245.

Romeo DM, Cowan FM, Haataja L et al. (2020) Hammersmith Infant Neurological Examination for infants born preterm: predicting outcomes other than cerebral palsy. *Dev Med Child Neurol* **63**: 939–946.

Spittle A, Orton J, Anderson PJ et al. (2015) Early developmental intervention programmes provided post hospital discharge to prevent motor and cognitive impairment in preterm infants. *Cochrane Database Syst Rev* 11:CD005495.

Stanley F, Blair E, Alberman E (2000) *Cerebral Palsies: Epidemiology and Causal Pathways*. London: Mac Keith Press.

Straathof L, Heineman KR, Hamer EG et al. (2020) Prevailing head position to one side in early infancy – a population-based study. *Acta Paediatr* **109**: 1423–1429.

Straathof L, Heineman KR, Hamer EG et al. (2021) Patterns of atypical muscle tone in the general infant population: prevalence and associations with perinatal risk and neurodevelopmental status. *Early Hum Dev*, epub ahead of print.

Super CM, Harkness S (2015) Charting infant development: milestones along the way. In: Jensen LA (ed.) *The Oxford Handbook of Human Development and Culture: An Interdisciplinary Perspective*. Oxford: Oxford Handbooks Online, doi: 10.1093/oxfordhb/9780199948550.013.6.

Thomas JC, Letourneau N, Campbell TS et al. (2017) Developmental origins of infant emotion regulation: mediation by temperamental negativity and moderation by maternal sensitivity. *Dev Psychol* **53**: 611–628.

Touwen BCL (1976) *Neurological Development in Infancy*. London: Heinemann Medical Books.

Touwen BCL (1990) Variability and stereotypy of spontaneous motility as a predictor of neurological development of preterm infants. *Dev Med Child Neurol* **32**: 501–508.

Volpe JJ (2009) Brain injury in premature infants: a complex amalgam of destructive and developmental disturbances. *Lancet Neurol* **8**: 110–124.

Wu Y-C, Bouwstra H, Heineman KR et al. (2020) Atypical general movements in the general Dutch population: prevalence over the last 15 years and associated factors. *Acta Paediatr* **109**: 2762–2769.

Yakovlev PL, Lecours AR (1967) The myelogenetic cycles of regional maturation of the brain. In: Minkowski A (ed.) *Regional Development of the Brain in Early Life*. Oxford: Blackwell, pp. 3–70.

Zwaigenbaum L, Penner M (2018) Autism spectrum disorder: advances in diagnosis and evaluation. *BMJ* **361**: k1674.

Index

Other titles from Mac Keith Press www.mackeith.co.uk

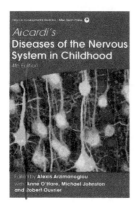

Aicardi's Diseases of the Nervous System in Childhood, 4th Edition

Alexis Arzimanoglou, Anne O'Hare, Michael V Johnston and Robert Ouvrier (Editors)

Clinics in Developmental Medicine
2018 ▪ 1524pp ▪ hardback ▪ 9781909962804

This fourth edition retains the patient-focussed, clinical approach of its predecessors. The international team of editors and contributors has honoured the request of the late Jean Aicardi, that his book remain 'resolutely clinical', which distinguishes *Diseases of the Nervous System in Childhood* from other texts in the field. New edition completely updated and revised and now in full colour.

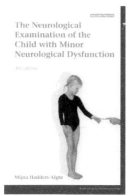

Neurological Examination of the Child with Minor Neurological Dysfunction, 3rd Edition
Mijna Hadders-Algra

Mac Keith Press Practical Guides
2010 ▪ 168pp ▪ softback ▪ 9781898683988

This highly practical book brings the examination of minor neurological dysfunction developed by Bert Touwen and his colleagues in Groningen right up to date, which is timely in view of the increasing interest in and use of this approach.
The approach is a detailed and extensive neurological examination with the aim of detecting a possible neurobiological basis for learning, behavioural and motor coordination problems in a child and thus informing decision-making and management. It provides a refined, sensitive and age-appropriate technique, designed to take into account the developmental aspects of the child,'s rapidly changing nervous system.

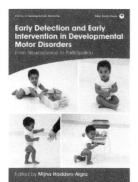

Early Detection and Early Intervention in Development Disorders: From Neuroscience to Participation
Mijna Hadders-Algra (Editor)

Clinics in Developmental Medicine
2021 ▪ 288pp ▪ hardback ▪ 9781911612438

The book provides a comprehensive overview of assessments and interventions applied in young children with or at high risk for developmental motor disorders. It provides an evidence-based practical guide for health professionals working in the field of early detection and early intervention.

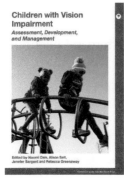

Children with Vision Impairment: Assessment, Development, and Management
Naomi Dale, Alison Salt, Jenefer Sargent, and Rebecca Greenaway (Editors)

Mac Keith Press Practical Guides
2021 • 288pp • softback• 9781911612339

Vision impairment is a long-term condition caused by disorders of the eye, optic nerve, and brain. Using evidence-based knowledge, theory, and research, this book provides practical guidance for practitioners who are involved in the care and management of children with long-term vision impairment and disability.

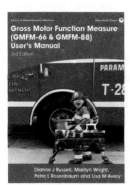

Gross Motor Function Measure (GMFM-66 & GMFM-88) User's Manual 3rd Edition
Dianne J Russell, Marilyn Wright, Peter L Rosenbaum, Lisa M Avery (Editors)

Clinics in Developmental Medicine
2021• 320pp • softback • 9781911612490

The third edition of the Gross Motor Function Measure (GMFM-66 & GMFM-88) User's Manual has retained the information contained in the original 2002 and 2013 publications which included the conceptual background to the development of the GMFM, and the administration and scoring guidelines for people to be able to administer this clinical and research assessment tool appropriately. The new edition contains updates and information on the GMFM App.

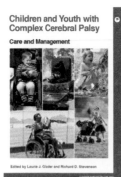

Children and Youth with Complex Cerebral Palsy: Care and Management
Maurie Glader & Richard Stevenson

Mac Keith Press Practical Guides
2018 • 404pp • softback • 9781909962989

Children with complex cerebral palsy (typically, but not always, GMFCS levels IV and V) require skilled management and extensive expertise which can be overwhelming or intimidating for many clinical practitioners. This book explores management of the many medical comorbidities these children encounter, including orthopedic concerns, mobility and equipment needs, cognition and sensory impairment, difficult behaviors, seizures, respiratory complications and nutritional challenges, among many others. In addition, adaptable care tools will be provided both in the text and as a resource to download from this page, to guide clinicians in evaluation, preventive care and crisis management.

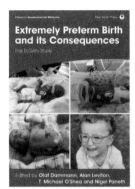

Extremely Preterm Birth and its Consequences: The ELGAN Study
Olaf Dammann, Alan Leviton, T Michael O'Shea, Nigel Paneth (Editors)

Clinics in Developmental Medicine
2020 ▪ 256pp ▪ hardback ▪ 9781911488965

The ELGAN (Extremely Low Gestational Age Newborns) Study was the largest and most comprehensive multicentre study ever completed for this population of babies born before 28 weeks' gestation. The authors' presentation and exploration of the results of the research will help clinicians to prevent adverse health outcomes and promote positive health for these children.

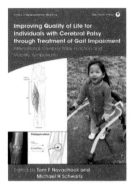

Improving Quality of Life for Individuals with Cerebral Palsy through Treatment of Gait Impairment
Tom Novacheck, Michael Schwartz (Editors)

Clinics in Developmental Medicine
2020 ▪ 163pp ▪ hardback ▪ 9781911612414

The *Symposium* brought together world-reknowned experts with a range of viewpoints to challenge each other and answer these questions, and prevent stagnation of outcomes. This publication unites these discussions to establish a framework to guide research efforts for the future and ensure meaningful progress. Authors consider how patient goals can be given more attention and ask how we can learn more details of the underlying neurological impairments.

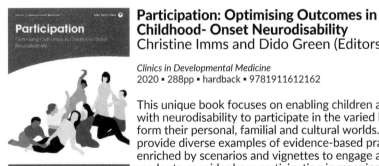

Participation: Optimising Outcomes in Childhood- Onset Neurodisability
Christine Imms and Dido Green (Editors)

Clinics in Developmental Medicine
2020 ▪ 288pp ▪ hardback ▪ 9781911612162

This unique book focuses on enabling children and young people with neurodisability to participate in the varied life situations that form their personal, familial and cultural worlds. Chapters provide diverse examples of evidence-based practices and are enriched by scenarios and vignettes to engage and challenge the reader to consider how participation in meaningful activities might be optimised for individuals and their families. The book's practical examples aim to facilitate knowledge transfer, clinical application and service planning for the future.

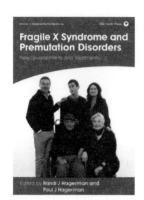

Fragile X Syndrome and Premutation Disorders: New Developments and Treatments
Randi J Hagerman, Paul J Hagerman (Editors)

Clinics in Developmental Medicine
2020 ▪ 192pp ▪ hardback▪ 9781911612377

Fragile X syndrome results from a gene mutation on the X-chromosome, which leads to various intellectual and developmental disabilities. Fragile X Syndrome and Premutation Disorders offers clinicians and families a multidisciplinary approach in order to provide the best possible care for patients with Fragile X. Unique features of the book include what to do when an infant or toddler is first diagnosed, the impact on the family and an international perspective on how different cultures perceive the syndrome.

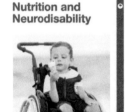
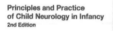

Nutrition and Neurodisability
Peter Sullivan, Guro Andersen, Morag Andrew (Editors)

Mac Keith Press Practical Guides
2020▪ 208pp ▪ softback ▪ 9781911612254

Feeding difficulties are common in children with neurodisability and disorders of the central nervous system can affect the movements required for safe and efficient eating and drinking. This practical guide provides strategies for managing the range of nutritional problems faced by children with neurodevelopmental disability.

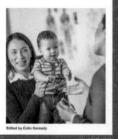

Principles and Practice of Child Neurology in Infancy, 2nd Edition
Colin Kennedy (Editor)

Mac Keith Press Practical Guides
2020 ▪ 552pp ▪ softback ▪ 9781911612001

Management of neurological disorders presenting in infancy poses many challenges for clinicians. Using a symptom-based approach, and covering a wide range of scenarios, the latest edition of this comprehensive practical guide provides authoritative advice from distinguished experts. It now includes revised coverage of disease prevention, clinical assessment, and promotion of neurodevelopment.